Second Edition

The **Ultimate Guide**
to **Trail Running**

Everything You Need to Know About

Equipment • Finding Trails • Nutrition • Hill Strategy •
Racing • Avoiding Injury • Training • Weather • Safety

Adam W. Chase and Nancy Hobbs

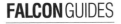

FALCON GUIDES

GUILFORD, CONNECTICUT
HELENA, MONTANA
AN IMPRINT OF GLOBE PEQUOT PRESS

FALCON GUIDES®

Project editor: David Legere
Text design: Sheryl P. Kober
Layout artist: Mary Ballachino

Illustrations on pages 102–7 and 109 are excerpted from Running Stretches poster, booklet, and handout sheet by Bob Anderson, illustrations by Jean Anderson, revised edition © 1997 Stretching Inc., and the revised edition of the book *Stretching* by Bob and Jean Anderson © 2000 Shelter Publications. Contact Stretching Inc. at P.O. Box 767, Palmer Lake, CO 80133-0767, www.stretching.com, or 1-800-333-1307 for a free catalog of Stretching Inc. publications/products.

Library of Congress Cataloging-in-Publication Data is available on file.

ISBN 978-0-7627-5537-0

Printed in the United States of America

10 9 8 7 6 5 4 3 2 1

ACKNOWLEDGMENTS

Our thanks to Noah and David Chase, Dr. James Hobbs, Peggy Whitney Hobbs, and Garry Harrington. We additionally thank those who contributed to the making of this text and to those who helped and inspired us in the writing of this book.

CONTENTS

FOREWORD

"Stuck in Laguna Beach and need a long run. Where would you go to put in 20 miles?" That was the e-mail I sent to Charlie Nickell. Snowstorms in New York were preventing me from getting home to Connecticut. I had been traveling on business as publisher of *Runner's World* and *Running Times* with the editors in chief of both magazines, David Willey and Jonathan Beverly. Following a meeting with Gary Slayton of Asics, we got the news that we were not going to make it home that night. Outstanding! I was training for Boston that winter, and now here I was in Southern California and could do my long run without freezing. But where?

I had met Charlie over the phone just weeks earlier. Charlie had been a successful but overweight executive who decided his type-A business regime would put him in an early grave. So he sold his business and went for a run. Being the overachiever, he went for a very, very long run, turning himself into a solid ultramarathoner and using his gift for writing to pen a regular blog (therundown.net) on his ultra exploits. Charlie had contacted me to see if he could submit a story to *RW*.

"I got a great run for you. Meet me at the corner of Santiago Road and Live Oak Canyon. Park in the lot next to the biker bar. 7 a.m. tomorrow. I'll bring bars, gels, and a hydration pack for you. Cool 16-mile trail run. If you need more, we'll give it to you!" This guy's good, I thought. But who is "we"? "See you then," I replied.

When I showed up, there were fifteen people waiting for me. But like Charlie, these weren't fifteen "normal" people. They were all members of the Orange County Trail Runners and all were accomplished trail runners and ultramarathoners. I was in big trouble. Charlie had sent an e-mail to the membership of the OCTR that "they had the chance to run with 'Running Royalty,' the publisher of *RW* is in town and wants to run with us!" Flattering maybe, but from that description it would seem like I was world class, fast and strong. Hardly. I would describe myself as a solid midpack runner. My running industry "friends" would describe me as a solid back of the packer. Maybe even a "penguin." As we all shook hands and then gathered for a pre-run photo, I couldn't help but notice how ripped and toned these guys and women were and how doughy that made me feel.

I was introduced to Michelle Barton. We chatted the kind of chat you have in a race corral. The difference, it turned out, is that I would be fifteen corrals behind Michelle. I learned from our little chat that she was the overall winner of the Twin Peaks 50K, got second in the Way Too Cool 50K and *won* the Javelina 100-Miler. Gulp. If I'm "running royalty," I'm their court jester. Michelle pointed up to the top of Santiago Peak— 5,600 feet above where we stood. "We're going up there." Oh my. Can I bail out now?

Wow. I couldn't imagine. Here I was trucking up a trail with fifteen amazing athletes, most of whom had trail runs over 100 miles under their belts. Twenty-two miles later and 11,200 feet gained and lost, we had experienced more than a long run. We came across an area where cattle rustlers in the 1800s hid out and watered their newly stolen property. Ironically, 10 miles later we ran out of water, a huge no-no, but because of my running partners' local knowledge, we found a trickling high-altitude aquifer (another trail running no-no as you'll find as you read on). We ran into other ultrarunners, the most impressive being sixty-six-year-old 100-miler veteran Hwa Ja Andrade, training solo by trekking 28 miles to the top of Santiago Peak and back! Otherworldly. All of us bonked at one point, but we all worked together to keep on. We saw amazing wildlife and incredible vistas high above the cloud layer all the way to the Pacific. Instead of running 16 miles, we were all so pumped we finished at the Tucker Wildlife Sanctuary having run 22.

That run embodied all that is great and tricky about trail running. While my experience with the OCTR was more than extreme, being on the trail is always an adventure regardless of how far you go. It's a full sensory experience. The sights, sounds, and smells are always amazing. There's no match for the camaraderie forged by the common experience of trail running. My regular run now is along the Del Mar Trail north to Torrey Pines State Park in California. It's pure bliss.

No runners are more qualified to co-author this book than Nancy Hobbs and Adam Chase. Period. Yes, they are a couple of the sport's best athletes with years and many miles of trails under their feet. But more so, it's their passion, enthusiasm, and unparalleled expertise for the sport and activity. They *are* trail running, and they will do all they can to get more people to safely experience what they have the privilege of doing every day.

I didn't think I could run with the likes of the OCTR. But like that adventure, this book will take you farther and to more beautiful places than you can imagine. Enjoy this book and the adventures it will open up to you. I hope you, too, have the misfortune of getting stuck in Laguna. Don't forget to call Charlie. You'll get more than you'd ever hoped for.

Andrew R. Hersam
Executive Vice President—Media
The Competitor Group
Former Publishing Director for *Runner's World* and *Running Times*
Running USA Board of Directors

PREFACE

I've been on all sorts of trails: long and short ones, mountain and desert, eastern to western, north to south, flat, steep, rocky, muddy, even paved trails. If a trail is not named, I'll give it one. I can recall trail names and their descriptions better than I can remember my PIN number. If I'm in one location long enough, I will cover all the trails in that area. If I'm driving and see a path meandering along, I wonder what it does when it twists out of view. I want to see where the trail goes, get to its highest point, and come back a different way. I like traveling light. I like to do in a single morning or afternoon what takes most people days. I love descending switchbacks on rocky scree fields and the feeling of my burning legs and lungs after a long climb. These things make me who I am. I am a trail runner.

On a recent run my breathing had become labored. I'd randomly decided that this was as far as I was going to go: 11,600 feet and relentless snowfields had brought me to a halt. I needed to dump the glacial till from my shoes, eat, and sip some water. The high sun would be upon me soon, and there were parts of me that were exposed and ripe for a burn. I stood in one of the many expansive cirques in the John Muir Wilderness Area on the eastern slope of the Sierras of California. I had left my truck two hours before and headed up the trail knowing only that retracing my steps would bring me back to my starting point. I hadn't seen another soul: Footprints from the last traveler had been washed away by the previous day's rain. This was what I was looking for.

Do you insist you don't sweat the small stuff: the traffic jams, the cranky bosses, the broken appliances, the neighbor's leaf blower, the plane overhead, a ringing cell phone, the bills to pay, a backlog of must-get-to e-mails, or even remembering where you last set your sunglasses? Each day you extend yourself. As you move through life you often dismiss day-to-day tribulations as minor. You feel you've grown accustomed to the small stressors. Any of these events by itself may not be so devastating, but their accumulation certainly is.

The human spirit and body perform in unison. The two are a package, one depending on the other. The healthiest individuals function well when the duo is in tip-top shape. In short, you generally have your best days when you are both content and healthy. Life's everyday hassles do, whether you know it or not, lessen your number of good days. So how do we rectify this situation? There are countless means to this end: medications, drugs, and therapy. However, the most utilitarian stress reliever is physical activity. I believe (and hope you'll agree) that trail running is the best approach to "curing what ails you."

The fact that you have picked up this book and have gotten as far as this preface is encouraging. You must have heard of the obvious benefits of trail running. Trails offer softer, varied terrain and enhance proprioception (one's body awareness in space), spare the body's joints, and provide a whole body workout. Trails also take you away from the dangers of vehicular traffic and the associated pollution they create.

However, let us not forget about the less tangible, almost mysterious, benefit of trail running, a benefit born from the environment where trails are found. The recuperative powers of a vegetative blind, the sounds of moving water, and fresh air and scenery not associated with our everyday surroundings have a significant positive impact on our psyche.

Whether your trail is located in the most remote wilderness in the country or found as easily as the greenway two blocks from your house, there is something curative about the natural space you have created around yourself. If only briefly you are reminded of what you need to do (inhale, lift your foot, move your arm) rather than what you believe you have to do (tend to your daily chores and duties), then you've been successful.

Trail running novices and veterans alike will benefit from what Nancy Hobbs and Adam Chase have put together here. This guide merges not only their own countless years of trail knowledge but also the wisdom of other greats in the sport as well. I think you'll find that *The Ultimate Guide to Trail Running* will help us all toward assembling our own collection of trails and their associated memories in a healthy and happy way.

Ian Torrence

INTRODUCTION

This is a "how to" book on trail running, written for runners of all abilities. With this second edition we hope to re-inspire readers of our first edition and welcome new readers to the trail running family. As the executive director and the president of the American Trail Running Association (ATRA), we have been asked by our members and others about how to begin trail running, what trails are best, what to wear and eat when trail running, how to train and race as a trail runner, how to organize a trail race, and a variety of other issues. The pleasure we receive in answering these questions and sharing our passion for the sport of trail running is what inspired us to write this book.

Through *The Ultimate Guide to Trail Running,* we hope to open the sport up to more people by equipping them with a wealth of information on all aspects of trail running. We hope that this book becomes a valuable resource for all trail runners, from the novice to the experienced, regardless of where they run. For those who have never run on anything other than a paved surface or a track and for hikers who have been on many a trail but never run on one, this book should provide enough information for anyone to get started running trails with a sense of competency.

This book should appeal to those with interests that include running trails to cross-country, fast hiking, recovering from overuse injuries or burnout from other sports including road running, training for adventure races or high school cross-country, competing in ultradistance trail races, or running entire trails such as the Appalachian, Muir Woods, or Continental Divide.

In writing this book, we have drawn on our combined experiences and solicited the advice and expertise of many contributors. It has been a rewarding experience to interview some of the top trail runners and experts in fields such as nutrition, sports physiology, environmental sciences, and even animal health. We have learned a lot while writing this book and hope to pass that knowledge on to you.

We begin *The Ultimate Guide to Trail Running* with a brief history and background of the sport. Next, we include instruction on trail-specific training, including basic trail technique, the effects of altitude, and how to strength train and stretch for trail running. We incorporate advice on how best to confront different types of trail conditions, such as mud, ice, water crossings, and steep hills. This section also weaves invaluable insights from experts or elite competitors who excel in running on various types of trails.

As a book for all types of runners, *The Ultimate Guide to Trail Running* addresses potential trail injuries and offers its readers specific advice from experts in sports medicine and the healing arts. We also provide a broad discussion of trail hazards, such as extreme weather, wildlife, dehydration, and safety concerns.

For the trail running gearhead, we include a survey of proper trail footwear, apparel, and accessories. There is also a section that discusses proper nutrition and expert advice on how to stay fueled and hydrated during your runs. We offer advice about running partners of all types: people, dogs, horses, burros, llamas, and children riding in all-terrain strollers.

The chapter on trail racing should entice the more competitive trail runner while providing valuable advice for race directors or future race directors on such topics as course marking, aid, bandits, and promotions. The checklists that accompany this section promise to be invaluable to any trail race organizer or competitor.

We could not write a book about trail running without focusing on the importance of environmental awareness. In the environmental section of the book, we address trail activism, trail etiquette, and how to coexist with multiple users, such as mountain bikers, horses, hikers, and dog walkers.

Throughout the text we incorporate some enjoyable trail tales—stories about the joy of trail running, including personal trail running and racing adventures. This sampling includes accounts of how runners "connect" with the sport and their environment, their spiritual insights, and other trail wisdom that contributors have chosen to pass on to you.

And now, by way of introduction, we include our own thoughts on trail running:

Nancy Hobbs

It's been almost ten years since the first edition of this book was published. It has been a full decade packed with trail runs and races in the United States and abroad. My passion for the sport has not waned, and each trail run leads me on a new adventure, whether I am alone or with friends. In addition to the myriad trails I enjoy, I still spend time running on the roads, usually getting to and from a trail, but I much prefer dirt, scree, and other natural obstacles underfoot as opposed to asphalt. Sharing a trail with a partner, especially a newcomer to the trails, further

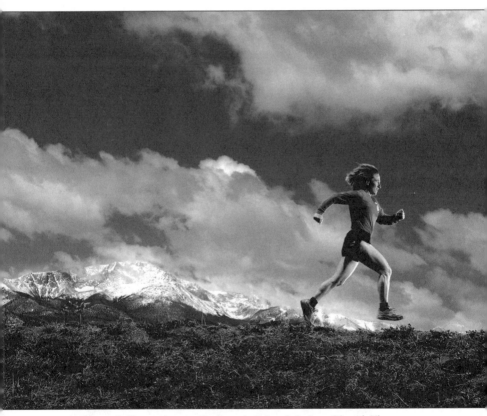

Author Nancy Hobbs running near her home in Colorado Springs, CO, with Pikes Peak in the background. Keith Ladzinski

enhances the experience. I have introduced many road runners to the joys of trail running and share their newfound enthusiasm as they tackle their first switchback or climb a steep grade to take in an expansive vista from the high point of a mountain.

You don't have to run too far along a trail to experience the peace, solitude, and scenic views inherent in this niche sport. And there will be days when though you're just a mile from the trailhead, you will meet the unexpected. I was twenty minutes into a training run in Franklin Canyon in the East Bay Regional Park system in Martinez, California, when my running partner Myles, a long-haired Weimaraner, spotted a furry friend on the trail ahead. Thinking it a squirrel, or a stray cat, I didn't worry as Myles went charging after the critter. As I got closer to watch the encounter unfold, the critter turned his back on Myles and sprayed a thick, syrupy yellow mass onto his face and shoulder. This not-so-flowery essence was overwhelming, as I quickly found out when Myles tried to take refuge by my side. I started running faster to escape the smell, but Myles stayed with me. Not only that, but the skunk's spray had also adhered to my clothes. After the run, I loaded Myles into the bed of the truck and headed to the grocery store for tomato juice. I scrubbed Myles thoroughly, but even after two tomato juice baths he still sported a lingering skunk odor.

I cannot predict whether or not you will encounter a wild animal—ferocious, or not so much—on your trail runs, but I guarantee that you will have an adventure. Be open to the experience and you'll understand why trail running has been my passion over the past twenty years, a passion to share with you in the following pages.

Adam W. Chase

After running more than seventy-five marathons and ultramarathons, I dropped out of my first race during a 100K run on paved 10K loops. It was my first race off trails in years and the knee problems I suffered made me promise myself that it would be the last. While I don't totally shun roads now, I heavily favor trails and have added more than thirty marathons and ultras since that incident. It is quite common to see road runners "graduate" to the trails, although it is also a growing trend among high school and college age runners to embrace off-road running.

When runners complain of overuse injuries, it's a safe bet to assume that they got hurt from running on roads. Pounding the pavement with little variation in stride or foot strike, mile after mile, just isn't natural. We're simply not made for logging big miles on the streets.

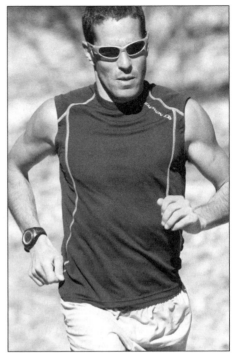

Author Adam W. Chase on trails of Mont Ventoux, France. Photo courtesy of Salomon, taken by Pierre Thomas

Granted, you will see some marvelous injuries as the result of trail running mishaps, but those trail injuries are typically of the more exciting flesh-wound category. It's so much more impressive to finish a trail race covered with dirt and dried streams of blood from skinned knees or elbows than it is to drop out of a road race because of an overworked iliotibial band or shin splint flare-up. Hell, you can't even see those!

The essence of trail running is the ability to deal with constant change. No two steps are the same on the natural obstacle course of off-road terrain. Even if you run the same trail day after day, you will soon learn that the trail has a life of its own. One day it may be dry and hard, the next it may be wet and sloppy. There are also the seasonal changes and the effects of temperature, erosion, foot traffic, and the (over)growth of plant life.

This constant change brings the running experience to life. Some of the best trail runners hail from a background of alpine or freestyle skiing or mountain biking. Like chess masters, talented trail runners exhibit an uncanny ability to always be three or four steps ahead of where their feet are at any given moment. This allows them to "set up" for turns, rocks, roots, or other variations that lie ahead, which is crucial to staying upright while maintaining downhill speed.

While there are literally hundreds of road running clubs throughout the United States, there are only a handful of trail running clubs. That fact speaks more to the type of people attracted to trail running than to the actual number of trail runners in this country. It highlights one of the differences that exist between road runners and trail runners. As a gross generalization, road runners are more likely to train in packs while trail runners gravitate more toward running solo. Perhaps road runners seek companionship out of the sheer boredom of the streets.

An accurate profile of a trail runner demands an in-depth analysis of the very psyche of those that identify themselves as trail runners. Just as the separation in the cycling world between "roadies" and mountain bikers is a distinction of attitude—as is the dichotomy between alpine skiers and telemarkers, sport and traditional climbers, triathletes and adventure racers, flat-water kayakers and white-water kayakers, track skiers and ski tour types—the difference between road runners and trail runners boils down to a psychological one.

The attitudinal distinction between a road runner and a trail runner is one between a quest for speed and distance versus pursuing something for an intrinsic, yet immeasurable, experience. Road runners tend to be into measurement. They are often aware of their pace and heart rate, the distance they have run, their personal record (PR) for that distance, and the calories they have burned. In contrast, while trail runners

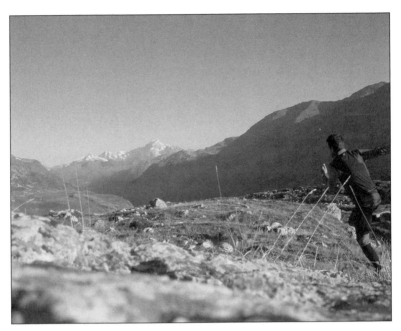

Jonathan Wyatt does some Alpine training. Jonathan Wyatt

might know the day of the week, they rarely know how far they have run, much less their pace, because they normally measure their runs by either time or distance, but not both.

The fact that roads are wide and trails narrow may help to explain why trail folk tend to be found in smaller numbers, but there is more to it. Trails offer the opportunity to retreat from the masses, to escape to a place of tranquility where your mind may wander without any concern for traffic. The distraction of having to scout each footstep can lull you into a peacefulness that cannot be found in a paved and populated environment.

Many more ultramarathons are run on trails than on roads. This is true for many reasons. First, the ultra community is a more mature crowd that has learned that the road to injury is paved, especially in races longer than 26.2 miles. Ultrarunners are also often characterized as aficionados of natural beauty, which is why the biggest and best ultras are run in some of the most awe-inspiring places, where runners are more likely to come across wildlife than they are vehicle traffic.

Trails are forgiving, especially if you are properly prepared for them, and I hope that *The Ultimate Guide to Trail Running* gives you that preparation.

CHAPTER 1

Trail Running:
Past, Present, and Future

It's difficult to say exactly where trail running originated. However, the United Kingdom is probably most deserving of the honor even though the term "trail" was not used initially to describe the activity. The first known hill race in the British Isles occurred sometime around 1068 in Scotland with the running of the legendary race to the top of Creag Choinnich at Braemar, a town about 75 miles north of Edinburgh. Robin Morris, member of the Scottish Hill Running Commission and race director for the 1995 World Mountain Running Trophy Race in Edinburgh, Scotland, summarizes the story as follows:

> King Malcolm II was known as Caen More or Big Head because he was full of good ideas. His kingdom was in need of a reliable system that could transfer information from place to place so Malcolm decided to establish a post system. The job interview took the form of a hill race.
>
> The hill chosen was the 1,764-foot Creag Choinnich, named by Kenneth II, who used it as a heading hill and lookout when his royal deer hunts took place in the valleys. The race began from the plain at 1,000 feet and would be won by the first runner to raise a standard at a point near the top that could be seen from the plain. The winning time was about three minutes and the champion received a baldric (a richly ornamented belt), a sword, and a purse of gold for his efforts.

Unfortunately, this first hill race did not survive. In 1842 the course was measured at 1,384 yards and was won in four minutes by James Cutts; but on September 12, 1850, the following account was recorded by Queen Victoria:

"We lunched early and then went to the Gathering at the Castle of Braemar. . . . There were the usual games of putting the stone, throwing the hammer and caber, and racing up the hill Creag Choinnich which was accomplished in less than six minutes and a half; and we were all much pleased to see our gillie [a male servant or guide] Duncan, who is an active, good-looking man, win. Eighteen or nineteen started; and it looked very pretty to see them run off in their different coloured kilts with their white shirts." She later added a footnote: "One of our keepers (the victor), like many others, spit blood after running up that steep hill. The running up the hill has consequently been discontinued." (The complete story is delightfully told by John Grant in his *Legends of the Braes O'Marr*.)

According to Douglas Barry of the Irish Mountain Running Association, trail running has been recorded in Ireland since pre-Christian times. Barry relates a piece of folklore: "When legendary Irish hero Fionn Mac-Cumhaill [Finn McCool] was getting old, the chief of the Fianna [heroes to a man and guardians of the high king of Ireland] decided to settle down and get married. With no dating agencies around, Fionn picked his future wife by staging a women-only race up and down Slievenamon Mountain in County Tipperary, which is Gaelic for "mountain of the women."

Deirdre, the very beautiful daughter of the local chief, won the race. Fionn was very pleased with the result. Unfortunately, the story didn't have a happy ending.

When Deirdre saw the rather wrinkly Fionn, she didn't fancy him at all. She ran away with Diarmuid—Fionn's younger lieutenant in the Fianna. This prompted a monumental chase that is recorded in the annals of ancient Ireland.

Many other mountain races were staged throughout Irish history, although the first event that made the record books was one held in 1873 on the Sugarloaf in County Wicklow. The race was organized by noted Irish climber and traveler Sir Charles Barrington, who in addition to owning the horse Sir Robert Peel, a winner of the Irish Grand National horse race, was the first man to climb Switzerland's Eiger in 1858. A man appropriately named Tom Hill was the first to cross the finish line, and he was awarded the coveted victor's prize, a gold watch donated by the wealthy Barrington.

Danny Hughes, president of the World Mountain Running Association (WMRA) from 1993 until his death in February 2009, often recited stories about mountain racing in England and its development from the practice of shepherds challenging one another to short races up and down the local fells, to professional mountain guide races in Victorian times. *Fell* is chiefly regarded as a Scottish term relating to mountain or height. In the British dialect, fell refers to an elevated wild field or a hill moor. Hills and mountains are known as fells in the north of England after the Norwegian word *fjell*, as a result of the Viking invasions of 1,000 years ago.

These races usually took place in conjunction with the local country shows and were known as Guides Races. The earliest records date back to the 1850s, the most famous of all being the Grasmere Guides Race, which has been run more or less consistently since 1868. The year 1895 saw the first race to the summit of Ben Nevis and back, a distance of 16 kilometers and 1,500 meters of ascent and descent. Ben Nevis is located in the Scottish highlands and is the highest mountain in Great Britain. It wasn't until as recently as 1995 that the so-called professional Guides Races and the amateur races became open to all comers as antiquated regulations were swept aside.

As evidenced by these century-old tales, the United Kingdom's long history in hill running is considered a predecessor of trail and mountain running. Over time the sport has become more organized, and in 1970 the Fell Running Association (FRA) was formed to cater to the needs of amateur hill runners. Today the FRA is recognized by UK Athletics as the managing body of individual athletes (5,000) as well as their athletic clubs. Wales, Scotland, and North Ireland have similar but smaller organizations responsible for the sport in their regions. The original purpose of the FRA was the distribution of a calendar of events, but later it inaugurated a newsletter and now glossy four-color magazine, *The Fell Runner,* and a hill racing championship. The annual fell-running calendar of events has grown from 40 events in 1970 to more than 500 in 2009. "The 2009 UK Race Calendar has 511 races, including 7, 33, and 52 from Northern Ireland, Scotland, and Wales respectively. This is probably about three-quarters of the races held in Wales annually but only about a quarter of those held in Scotland. The number of races continues to increase every year. There are probably a lot more held in England as well that do not appear in the calendar," according to Adrian Woods, Welsh National event coach and runner.

The Fell Runner is currently published three times per year, and annual championships consisting of points awarded for the best results from several races are staged in each region and in the United Kingdom as a whole.

The European (Continental) style of trail running is strongly oriented toward uphill courses rather than the uphill/downhill versions so prevalent in the United Kingdom. Numerous trail and mountain races exist in Europe, many being held at popular ski areas. The European events are very well supported in terms of participants, spectators, and the media, and the courses are always challenging, with a variety of running surfaces encountered throughout the race.

It is difficult to pinpoint the precise time that trail and mountain running developed in the United States. Games that were established during colonial times certainly included elements of trail running, which provided a forum for competition. American history combined with European and British folklore have, over time, created what is now a growing sport in the United States, with both uphill and uphill/downhill venues being equally represented. Race distances range from 1 mile to ultradistances of more than 26.2 miles. Races exist for every type of trail runner—from the recreational athlete to the elite-level competitor, and from the short-distance athlete to the ultradistance enthusiast.

DEFINING THE SPORT OF TRAIL RUNNING

The definition of *trail* can vary widely, from paved nonmotorized pathways that run parallel to city streets or flank city parks, to tracks made by animals passing through a remote wilderness region, to footpaths designed by officials within state, regional, or national parks. Because this book is dedicated to the wilder, more adventurous side of trail running, the unpaved trail will be our focus. This is not to say that paved pathways are void of adventure; they just don't provide the same sort of experience that one encounters when running unpaved trails.

Trail running terrain can vary widely within and between regions across the United States and can also change dramatically from season

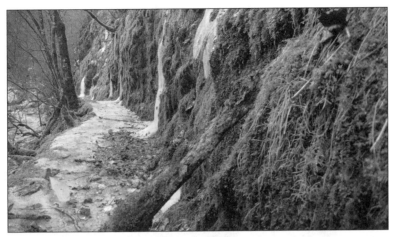

Trails afford challenges underfoot and unlock the beauty of our natural resources.
Stephan/Gripmaster

to season. For instance, much of the trail running in California is on fire roads in regional and state parks, although numerous singletrack trails also exist, many of which are interspersed with the fire roads. What can be dry and crackling underfoot in the summer can turn to mud and slop in the wetter months of winter and early spring. On the East Coast, it is common to run on trails laden with tree roots, multicolored leaves, and rocks. In Hawaii, forested areas that receive incredible rainfall often create a muddy surface that is as slick as an oiled pig. Switchbacks occur more frequently on the steeper mountain trails, and footing is usually more difficult on the heavily rock-strewn terrain at higher elevations. Of course, natural obstacles can occur just about anywhere one encounters running water, steep slopes, forest, rocks, or some combination of these features.

The majority of the trails referenced in this book will have at least three of the four following characteristics. They will: (1) be unpaved; (2) have natural obstacles that may include but are not limited to rocks, tree stumps, tree roots, dirt, gravel, mud, moraine, leaves, ice, snow, and creek crossings; (3) have a significant gain or loss of elevation; (4) include scenic vistas. Some mountain races described in this book include a portion or an entire route on pavement; however, these races do provide scenic

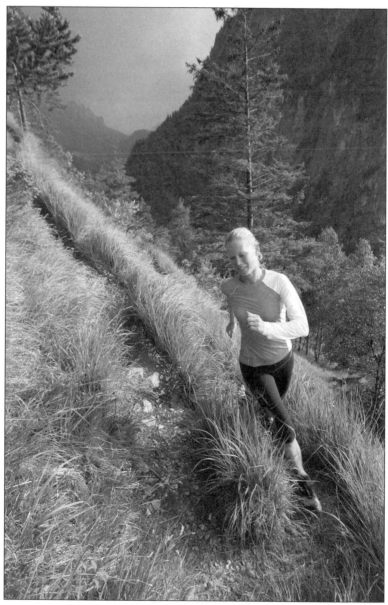

Christine Lundy, Team USA, at the World Mountain Running Championships 2009 in Italy.
Nancy Hobbs

vistas, significant elevation gain or loss, and often have some natural obstacles such as falling rock, downed trees, or potholes.

Trail running and mountain running are often used interchangeably in discussions and on Web sites referencing the activity. Sometimes the commingling of the terms is relevant and appropriate. For example, running in the mountains on nonpaved surfaces can be referred to as either mountain or trail running. However, running up Colorado's Mount Evans on the highway—the highest paved road in North America—can be called mountain running, but it should not be referred to as trail running, because it is on a paved surface open to motor vehicles. Likewise, the Mount Washington Race held in Gorham, New Hampshire, is considered a mountain run, even a "hill climb," since it involves only uphill running. The gravel surface of the route permits vehicular traffic and has an average grade of 11 percent over the 7.6-mile route, providing a significant enough elevation gain to be classified as a mountain run. This event is extremely popular, and with the 50th running in 2010, a Mount Washington Road Racing Hall of Fame will induct its first Hall of Fame class.

To add clarification, trail and mountain running have been categorized using several elements that include terrain/surface, elevation (gain or loss), and distance. The following descriptions better define the terms.

Mountain Running: The major component in mountain running is elevation gain or loss and may include steep ascents or descents. Surface, distance, and terrain further define mountain running. For example, a mountain run can be on paved surfaces, so long as significant elevation change (ascending) is present. The World Mountain Running Championships is recognized as the annual international event for this discipline. Since 2004 the WMRA has also held the World Long Distance Challenge for individual and team competition held in conjunction with a major mountain race; in 2010 the Pikes Peak Ascent (Manitou Springs, Colorado) will host the event. Each year since 2003, USA Track & Field (USATF) has staged a mountain running championship event. There is also a regional mountain running team championship contested by the North American Central American Caribbean (NACAC) member federations.

Trail Running: The major component in trail running is the nonpaved surface. Terrain can vary widely including grass, mud, rock, sand, gravel, scree, and snow, possibly with natural obstacles such as tree roots and water crossings. Trails can be any length or distance. Internationally recognized trail running championship events were instituted by the International Association of Ultra Runners (IAU) in 2005 with the now-defunct Sunmart 50-Mile Trail Race as the host in 2006 and 2007. There was no host in 2008, but in 2009 the IAU Trail Championships were held in Serre Chevalier, France. USATF has hosted national trail running championships at 10 kilometers, marathon, 50 kilometers, 50 miles, 100 kilometers, and 100 miles. The events are coordinated by the Mountain Ultra Trail (MUT) Council under the direction of the long distance running division within USATF. Information about bidding for a national championship is available at www.usatf.org.

Fell Running: A fell race is one run on fell, hill, or mountain terrain. The Fell Running Association (FRA) provides categories for races determined by vertical climb per mile, percentage on road, and length. Race length divides fell running into three categories: long (more than 12 miles), medium (6 to 8 miles), and short (less than 6 miles). Each constituent country in the United Kingdom held its own national championship—England, Scotland, Wales, and Northern Ireland—until 2009 when the UK was represented by one team at the 25th World Mountain Running Championships in Italy.

Additional Types of Running

Cross-Country: The major component is terrain further defined by distance (events typically range from 3 to 12 kilometers) and course width (at least 20 feet wide), with the focus on team-oriented competitions. Cross-country runs are similar to trail runs because both occur on non-paved surfaces. However, cross-country, unlike trail running, which is more of a free-form sport, has specific rules and guidelines set forth by USATF regarding the design of race courses, race distance, and competition criteria. Stipulations include the avoidance of very high obstacles, deep ditches, dangerous ascents or descents, thick overgrowth, and any obstacle that would constitute a difficulty beyond the aim of competition. One international event, the IAAF World Cross Country Championships, is held annually and is supported by the International Association of Athletics Federations (IAAF). In the United States, cross-country is a sport council within the long distance running division of USATF.

Skyrunning: The major component in Skyrunning is altitude. All Skyrunning events occur at elevations at or above 6,000 feet or 2,000 meters. Skyrunning includes the SkyMarathon (covering the full marathon distance reaching 14,000 feet or about 4,200 meters) and the SkyRace (which can be longer or shorter than the marathon and must reach at least 9,800 feet or 3,000 meters). The Vertical Kilometer, as its name suggests, has a vertical climb of 1,000 meters (3,048 feet) at various altitudes with variable distance according to the terrain (approximately 3 to 5 kilometers long). Terrain, elevation changes, and distance further define Skyrunning. Conducted by the International Skyrunning Federation, the 2009 Skyrunner World Series included sixteen races in fourteen countries across four continents with 6,000 competitors from thirty-one countries. The Skyrunner World Series is an annual series and is open to individual Skyrunners and commercially sponsored teams based on the sum of the best three World Series' race results and one World Series Trial.

Ultrarunning: Ultrarunning's major component is a distance beyond the marathon (26.2 miles). Ultraruns are further defined by terrain such as trails in the mountains or paved surfaces. The international championship event is the IAU World Cup 100K, which is held on paved roads. The IAU added a 50-kilometer event to its schedule in 2009.

Hashing: Although hashes, as the races are called, can be held on paved surfaces, the preferred terrain is trail or "shiggy." Hash runners include "hares" and "hounds." The hare(s) set out first, laying a flour-marked trail either as a dead hare (pre-laid) or a live hare (laid day of event) trail. The hounds follow the markings from a designated start point to the eventual finish line. The object of the hash is for the hounds to snare the hare before reaching the finish line, usually a one- to two-hour journey over a 3- to

5-mile course. The sport officially began in Kuala Lumpur in 1938 and has grown to more than 1,500 chapters worldwide, with the majority of clubs open to men and women of all ages and abilities. Though there is no official governing body, there are a few hash "traditions" that are loosely followed throughout the world. Hash traditions exist so a club can establish a starting point from where individual hash traditions evolve.

Other off-road running categories require distinctive equipment. These include **snowshoe running,** the major component being a snow-covered surface that is further defined by terrain, elevation, and distance, and **burro racing,** which requires a competitor to lead a burro fitted with a pack saddle and traditional mining equipment from start to finish. Burro racing is further defined by distance, terrain, and elevation changes. **Ride & Ties** include a pair of competitors who alternate riding a horse and running from start to finish (one competitor runs while the other competitor rides) and are further defined by terrain and distance. The object is to cover the course (ranging from 20 to 50 miles) in as short a time as possible by running or riding the entire distance. The distance between ties is solely determined by the team members.

Orienteering and **rogaining** (Rugged Outdoor Group Activity Involving Navigation and Endurance) utilize a detailed map and compass to locate points on the landscape.

Orienteering competition is always conducted with individual participation, awarding both age group and overall prizes for finishing with the fastest time over a predesignated course. Competitors normally start at two-minute intervals to reduce the potential for following another's route. Distances are usually between 4 and 12 kilometers with winning times ranging from thirty minutes to two hours, roughly six to eight minutes per kilometer. There are no markings to show the way, rather control points along the course that must be visited in sequence. At these points the competitors must record their presence by either punching a card or scanning a chip they carry with them. "Orienteering is a sport where you must enjoy at least two of the following—being in the woods, running, or reading maps. To excel, you must enjoy and be good at all three," said multi–age group champion Tony Federer, who has competed for the past thirty-four years in this sport. "Fortunately I am really good at reading maps, and I started spending more time running on the trails to further improve my results, and of course I love being out in the woods."

Rogaining competitions are held on courses that are not predetermined; rather, the participants choose their own route to maximize the number of points they can accumulate throughout a time period of six, twelve, or twenty-four hours. Each control point carries a different "score," with the farthest points and the more difficult to navigate garnering the highest point values. There are time penalties assessed for not reaching the finish line in the designated time period. Rogaining requires pre-planning, which is included in your cumulative finish time. Two-person teams compete for awards. Divisions may include female, male, or mixed further designated by age groups.

Adventure races created yet another niche. Many adventure races include a mountain or trail running leg, as do popular mountain bike "off-road" duathlons and triathlons.

GOVERNANCE

The disciplines outlined above each have an organizing body that oversees the conduct of their sport.

USA Track & Field

Cross-country running, mountain running, trail running, and ultrarunning are all organized sports within the long distance division of USA Track & Field (USATF).

Cross-country running was united under the long distance running division of USATF as a sport council in 2000. Prior to that time, men's cross-country was included in long distance running and women's cross-country was under the purview of track and field.

The Mountain Ultra Trail (MUT) Council formed in 1998 (as a subcommittee earning council status in 2000) to address the needs of elite-level competitors on the international level as well as to develop grassroots running programs throughout the United States. The MUT Council is comprised of representatives from women's, men's, and master's long distance running, as well as representatives from each USATF member association.

American Trail Running Association

The nonprofit Colorado-based American Trail Running Association (ATRA) was formed in 1996 to represent and promote the sport. ATRA is a national, membership-based organization that holds annual meetings to discuss current trends and issues in the sport. The group has a Web site, www.trailrunner.com, and produces a quarterly e-newsletter, *Trail Times*. ATRA is a member organization of USATF, Road Runners Club of America (RRCA), International Skyrunning Federation (ISF), and Running USA. ATRA coordinates all of the sponsorship and fund-raising for the national mountain running team.

American Ultrarunning Association

The American Ultrarunning Association (AUA), based in Morristown, New Jersey, was formed in 1990 to develop and promote ultrarunning (racing beyond the 26.2-mile distance) in the United States. It is a national member organization of USA Track & Field. AUA is an advocacy group for American ultrarunners, with emphasis on disseminating information and networking among ultrarunners, race directors, and corporate sponsors; developing opportunities for athletes; and promoting ultradistance events.

International Skyrunning Federation

Skyrunning falls under the purview of the International Federation for Skyrunning, which was founded in 2008 following the transformation of the Federation for Sport at Altitude (FSA), founded in 1995. The International Skyrunning Federation was created to promote, govern, and administer the sport of Skyrunning and similar multisports activities. For details on qualifying for Skyrunning events, please see the appendix.

Even though these organizations address the needs associated with the sport of trail running, many individuals choose to run trails on their own time and in their own space, preferring to remain anonymous, independent, and unorganized.

CHAPTER 2

Getting Started

Trail runners share common traits regardless of the number of miles or amount of time they've put into their off-road experiences. These include a desire for adventure and challenge, love of the outdoors, and an interest in communing with nature. Most who give the sport a try are hooked the first time out.

Tom Sobal has been running trails for years in and around his home in Salida, Colorado. "Trail running is an activity that can be done on virtually any trail, whereas certain other modes of transportation such as horseback riding or bicycling are not feasible on some trails due to severe obstacles such as large rocks, very steep terrain, steps, etc. Trail runners can easily modify their pace, foot plants, and movements to overcome an obstacle and quickly return to a more normal running motion without interrupting the flow of a run. Other modes of transport tend to restrict themselves to certain trails. Overcoming certain obstacles requires a dismount for other forms of transport, and too many of these interrupt those activities enough so that those users avoid certain trails."

Trail runners come in all shapes and sizes and may never have run a step before venturing onto trails. Although an athletic background is more common, it is far from a prerequisite.

Annette Bednosky started trail running the summer after she graduated from college. "I worked in Yosemite National Park as a Valley tour guide. During my days off I'd take off into the backcountry for long day hikes, usually solo because none of my friends wanted to go far. I wore running shoes as I did not own hiking boots (or a headlamp). Several times I wound up running the last few miles in the dusk just to get back to the trailhead before dark. By the end of the summer I was running the trails of Yosemite on purpose in order to cover more beautiful miles. My new habit stuck!"

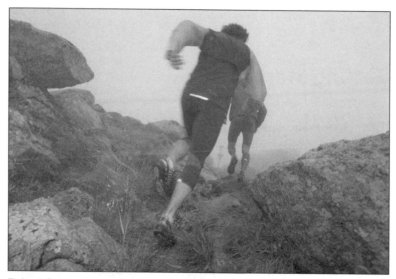

Trying to keep pace on an ascent can double the challenge. Stephan/Gripmaster

A similar story comes from Tim Dallas, who was a park ranger in Yosemite from 1978 to 1984. He sometimes had to move quickly over long distances during search and rescue operations. When he later moved to the San Francisco Bay Area, he started running and racing regularly to stay in shape, but soon decided being out in wilder terrain was more enjoyable, and running was more about being out on the trails and more than just exercise.

Laura Clark began running trails in 1976 while living in Heidelberg, Germany. "I discovered Volksmarching, or 'people's walk,' a popular weekend activity. Every town would host several per year and it was an excellent way to see the countryside. I hooked up with some German guys who liked to run these and received my first introduction to trail running."

Many road runners migrate to the softer surfaces of the trails because they hope to avoid impact injuries common to running on hard surfaces such as macadam or concrete. Once on the trail, road-shock trauma often subsides. Mike Teger, an aerospace engineer in Colorado Springs, enjoys most outdoor sports and tried running a few times on paved roads many years ago. "It was hard on my knees and about as interesting as grass grow." Teger then tried trail running and found that not trails kinder to his knees but they're also a lot more interesting. asphalt and concrete with dirt and rocks, monotonous homes and storefronts with lush alpine fields and towering pine trees, and barking dogs with marmots and pikas—what a world of difference!"

Athletes with varied sports backgrounds have also become trail runners. Phil Hadley, a former ski racer, became a trail runner while living in Boulder, Colorado. A friend took him out to Dakota Ridge where Hadley discovered he was in good enough shape (from road running) to run hilly trails. For Hadley, trail running combines his love of mountains and hiking with a competitive spirit that remains from his ski-racing days.

Paul Bateson was racing cyclocross in the '70s, and trail running fit into his training. Brandy Erholtz, USATF Mountain Runner of the Year 2008, first started running trails in college, heading out on the trails on easy days to cut down on some of the pounding. Aspen, Colorado, resident Rickey Gates started running cross-country in high school, and his coach, Mark Barbour, would take the team to one of the many trails in the area every Wednesday during the season. "Those were my fondest memories from high school—running East Maroon Trail in September when the aspen leaves were golden and I was with most of my closest friends."

Paul Charteris started trail running in 2006 primarily to train for triathlons because "I was an awful runner." Before he started running, Charteris hiked the same trails for two months. Every weekend he would do a long hike, which helped build up his legs and cardio output so that when he started running he was more prepared for the transition.

For Oregonian Carl Sniffen, trail running was a way to cross train for road and track racing. "I trail ran to develop foot and ankle strength and get stronger on the hills."

Beverley Anderson-Abs started running trails to train for adventure racing after watching the Eco-Challenge. When her team got a spot in Eco-Challenge Borneo, they hit the trails much more. As Anderson-Abs got stronger and faster in trail running and ultramarathons, she gradually shifted her focus to ultras and now only does an adventure race periodically.

New Yorker David Wise started running trails in the mid '80s. "As my kids were coming along I had less time for team sports. I became more serious about running, which up to that point had been solely recreational. Fortunately there are lots of trails near my home and I began to frequent them to get away from motorists. Trail running has become my favorite form of running."

Those who live in areas boasting trails find the sport a natural fit. Jim Tabb got hooked on trail running while living in Bishop, California—the amazing "east side" of the Sierra Nevada. Tabb says, "Slam dancing with Mother Nature on the east side is nothing short of magic. My back door has led me to encounters with mountain lions, thunderstorms, fresh air, and the most dramatic views in the world. How could I not get snagged."

Trail runners are year-round participants who can enter the sport at any time. Matthew Lewallen, a civil engineer from Denver, became obsessed with trail running during a run in the rugged mountains of Wyoming. "I was at an elevation of about 7,500 feet and the wind was blasting through the trees so hard I couldn't hear my own breathing. About five inches of virgin snow was on the ground and for a moment it seemed surreal. I took pride that I could conquer the elements with only my legs, some running shoes, and my own will to achieve."

Boulder couple Ryan and Lori Cooper enjoy their trail runs together and find they can usually cover distances comparable to two-day backpacking trips in one long run, enabling them to see the wilderness more quickly and easily without the added weight of a heavy pack. According to the pair, "This is not to infer that we don't take in the beauty; we just do it in an accelerated mode."

Courtney Johnson started running trails when she moved to Boulder in 1999, but from 2000 to 2004 while working full time in graduate school, she didn't have time to run. "Soon after my sister passed away unexpectedly, I found that trail running helped me to heal and refreshes my spirit and outlook on life."

Pam Pedlow started running trails when she was in her early twenties, "around 1975 . . . you do the math," says Pedlow. "Thanks to the influence of Jim Fixx, I started running, but was too self-conscious to run on the roads so I chose to run along the trails of the canyon. The solitude and the peace of my surroundings helped me review study notes and/or de-stress from work. By the time I came home I felt relaxed and refreshed."

Terry Chiplin and his wife, Jacqui, traveled 4,000 miles from England to follow their dreams—to establish a residential retreat, training, and active vacation center in Estes Park, Colorado. "We both loved running—in fact we met and fell in love at a running club in Bristol, England; our first 'date' was a 10-mile run! The clean air, the climate, and the majestic scenery in Colorado had drawn us like an irresistible magnet from afar—we hadn't reckoned on the trails though. I had been a road runner back in England. Soon after moving to Estes Park I became a trail runner. Trails were taking us to places we had never been before, and connecting us to the environment and our spirituality in a way that road running had never been able to. We started 'dancing' on the trails. Running became an opportunity to dance along the trails, skipping from rock to rock, or side to side, playing excitedly with the terrain like a long lost lover."

Hatchet Job

By Don Kardong

It had been a hard winter in Spokane, with a record snowfall of nearly 100 inches. Those conditions meant my favorite trail was inaccessible for months, and it wasn't until the end of March that I finally ventured back. Even then there were large patches of slush to maneuver through, but at least I was back doing what I love best—trail running.

The trail showed clear signs of winter battle fatigue. Dozens of branches had snapped off and fallen across the path, which was to be expected. But I was stunned at one point to find an ancient Douglas fir, nearly 3 feet in diameter, which had been uprooted by its burden of snow and had collapsed across the trail. I gingerly scuttled up and over. That, I surmised, was going to be an obstacle to trail users like myself for years to come.

I missed the following week's run, but the week after that, as I approached the fallen tree again, I noticed something odd. Someone had begun hacking into the beast with a hatchet. Wood chips were strewn on the ground, and the hatchet was stuck in the tree near the cut, with a lightweight chain attached to the handle. The other end of the chain was imbedded in the tree.

Who, I wondered, had left the hatchet there, and why? Were they planning to return periodically to use it? Did someone really expect to cut through the trunk of the massive conifer one chop at a time? Who would even own a hatchet with a chain attached?

Weird. I wondered about this during the rest of my run.

A week later, approaching the tree again, I stopped. The hatchet was still there. This time, though, the cut in the tree was twice as deep. I paused. Okay, I thought, count me in. I pulled the hatchet loose and gave the cut a hundred whacks. It didn't make much of a dent, but progress often comes one chip at a time. If I did this every time I came through here—if everyone who came through whacked the trunk a few times—eventually, months later, we might actually cut our way through.

So that's what I did, each week. One hundred whacks on the way out. One hundred whacks on the way back. I never saw anyone else chopping, but I knew they'd been there. In an incredibly short period of time—unbidden by anyone and anonymous to each other—we trail users made it halfway through.

About then I developed an Achilles pain that required a break from running. When I returned to the trail three weeks later, I was eager to find out how much progress my anonymous trail mates had made. Had they finally chopped through?

Imagine my disappointment then, when I approached the tree and saw that someone had sliced through the trunk with a chainsaw. The hatchet was gone. Yes, the trail was now clear, and if this had been done in the beginning, who could have objected? Instead, the clean cut had ruined the fun for an unspecified number of unidentified trail users, all of whom had shared the same unspoken goal.

So who scuttled our hard work and determination? Like so much else in this episode—like so much that happens out on the trail—I suspect the answer to that will remain a mystery. But each time I pass that spot on the trail, I can't help but taste the sour bile of disappointment.

A SPORT FOR EVERYONE

While trail running is a sport for people of all ages, it has appealed more to an older population, especially when looking at race results. (This may be due in part to a mandatory age of eighteen for some events.) Typically more men enter races than women, although the percentage difference has decreased from more than 80 percent men twenty years ago to a current average of about 68 percent men. Some races reflect an even split between male and female competitors, but this is rare.

In some European races and even some races in the United States, prize money may be a contributing factor in this inequity when the purse is less for women than men. Several arguments are advanced for and against this disparity. One side states that women don't have as much depth or representation so they should not have or expect equal prize money. On the other hand, top females train and work just as hard as do top males, so they should have an opportunity to race for equal prizes.

It has become clear over the years that race statistics may not accurately reflect the number of women who participate in trail running, perhaps because some avoid the competitive atmosphere associated with races, while others are simply not encouraged to race. These factors may be equally true of men. One way to provide encouragement and growth for the sport for both sexes is to emulate Bill Smith, a trail race director from Lancaster, Pennsylvania. Smith provides a venue that is supportive for the athlete who wants to enter an event and feel comfortable and welcome, surrounded by his or her peers. Smith stages a women-only trail race each Mother's Day and a men's-only race on Father's Day.

Another method that race directors use to encourage new trail runners is to identify them during a pre-race meeting or at the start line. When first-timers are asked to raise their hands, their more-experienced

ı the crowd cheer them on, usually to the first of many trail
s to come.

ɔldsmith, two-time USATF Mountain Runner of the Year says:
"Iraıı .. ıing requires such an athletic style of running that a lifelong
athlete will probably adapt better, say someone who has soccer or
some agility sport in their background of experience. That said, I think
it behooves a beginning trail runner to do some agility-type training
regularly along with their running training. I am talking about anything
from jumping rope to jump squats, running stairs, bounding, skipping,
high knee drills, butt kicks; exercise that trains you to lift your feet off
the ground with quickness. And, I would remind the runner to not run
exclusively on trails as running dirt roads or even on pavement will keep
leg speed (rapid turnover) in the muscle memory. As for racing, I say 'just
do it!' In all sports, I find racing and competing raises my level of skill
and helps me to find my true edge; racing is where breakthroughs are
discovered."

No matter what your running or athletic background may be, the
best introduction to trail running is to pick a nice day, find a beautiful
gently rolling trail that offers dependable footing, and set off on a relaxed
run. Take walking breaks as often as necessary and allow yourself to be
carried away by the sounds of the natural environment and the peaceful
surroundings. As you move along at a steady and easy pace, absorb the
views and breathe the clean air. From your initial experience gradually
build your running fitness and develop your trail running technique and
skills. This chapter will introduce you to these skills.

FINDING THE TRAILS

Living in the mountains is not a prerequisite for an aspiring trail runner.
In fact, many urban areas boast trail systems that delight and satisfy
trail runners of all levels. Finding trails requires little effort beyond a few
phone calls or a visit to the Internet.

Local and National Park Systems

Many cities and counties have local parks departments, which are wonderful resources. Consult the government section of the phone book or

visit the Internet for contact information. Additionally, the USDA Forest Service provides a complete listing of public areas with trail access, as does the National Park Service. Be sure to check the availability of maps for purchase. Running friends who have already incorporated trail running into their lifestyle can also provide a listing of trails. Finding trails through exploration is an adventurous option. Remember to steer clear of golf courses or private lands unless you have gained express permission from owners. Refrain from crossing fenced areas and those posted NO TRESPASSING.

Clubs, Running Stores, and Social Networking

Your local YMCA, health club, or sporting goods shop will often have information on trails available, and many provide maps. Specialty running stores and running clubs provide information about places to run, and they often schedule weekly trail runs that anyone is welcome to attend. Check out local and regional trail race calendars, attend a race as a volunteer or spectator, and mingle with the participants post-race to get information about other trails in the area. Join a Facebook group, navigate through running blogs, and check out running-specific Web sites. It is easy to connect with friends and make new acquaintances on the myriad of social networking sites available to anyone with access to a computer.

Commute to the Trail

Since few of us live next to or near a trailhead, you may be resigned to running on the roads during the week and running on trails on the weekend, when a commute to and from a trail makes the experience more workable. Keep in mind: Non-proximity to a trail or infrequent trail running doesn't make one runner any less serious than another who logs all or the majority of his or her weekly miles on the trails.

ASSESSING YOUR FITNESS

When beginning any new fitness program, it is advisable to first visit a doctor for a complete physical to determine if any limitations to exercise exist. If your current fitness is limited to dog walking, casual strolling around the block, and little cardiovascular activity, begin a trail running program that intersperses short hikes with light jogging and include the cross-training exercises found in Chapter 4.

For runners and individuals approaching trail running from other cardiovascular activities, use time as a guide when starting a trail running program rather than distance. For example, if your current running program consists of three miles every other day, translate those miles into minutes and head for the trails, concentrating on that time as a goal. Don't worry that the distance may not be equivalent. Increase trail runs using minutes or hours as a guide rather than distance. Below is a good basic four-week plan if you are a beginning trail runner.

Beginning Trail Runner— A Four-Week Plan

Week One: M/W/F—20–30 minutes of walk/jog; Saturday or Sunday: 30 minutes of walk/jog

Week Two: M/W/F—20–30 minutes of walk/jog; Saturday or Sunday—30–40 minutes of walk/jog

Week Three: M/W/F—30–35 minutes of walk/jog; Saturday or Sunday—35–45 minutes of walk/jog

Week Four: M/W/F—30–40 minutes of walk/jog; Saturday or Sunday—45 minutes to 1 hour of walk/jog

Increase the amount of time spent jogging as comfort level permits. It is okay to walk!

• Tuesdays and Thursdays should be used for rest or light exercise.

• For those already in a cardiovascular fitness program, add more workouts each week and increase the exercise times based on the workload you are comfortable with but not more than 10 percent per week. Weekend runs can be significantly longer than those listed above.

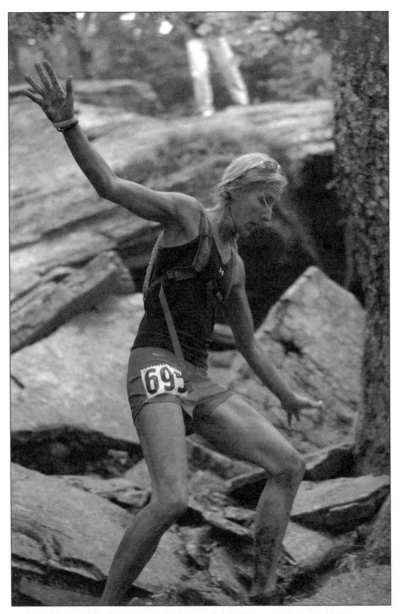

Michelle Roy navigates the route at the Escarpment Trail Race. Garry Harrington

HOW TO HANDLE THE HILLS

For the uninitiated, simply running trails presents enough of a challenge. When you're just starting out, there is no need to throw hills into the mix until you've achieved a level of comfort dealing with uneven footing on a level plain. Just as trail running works different muscles than does road running, hill running—both ascents and descents—can put a tremendous amount of strain on untrained muscles. Thus, trail neophytes should be prudent about introducing rougher trails into their trail-training routines.

Once you've achieved a level of confidence and competence running flat trails to the point where you are comfortable when confronting obstacles such as dirt, rocky terrain, fallen branches, mud, snow, and ice, then it is time to graduate to inserting some vertical into the running. There are two methods by which to introduce hills into your training regimen. The two should be treated as mutually exclusive, although it's okay to alternate them on different days; just don't integrate both on the same day—at least during the initial training stages.

Steep Grade/Stable Footing

The first method of hill training is to find a hill with a significant grade and stable footing. A steady climb and descent on a relatively steep dirt road serves as excellent training to condition muscles for hilly trail running. Depending on your fitness level, strength, athletic background, running goals, the length of the hill, the altitude, and other factors, a hill training session may involve repeats of running uphill for a minute or two and then walking for a minute, trading off between the two for fifteen to twenty minutes. When you reach the top, turn around and descend back to the start at a moderate pace. Alternatively, the repeats could integrate running uphill for a minute or two and then jogging down to start again for between four to seven repetitions.

Gradual Grade/Unsteady Footing

The second hill-running method is to pick a more gradual incline on a trail with less stable footing. Running longer repeats at a comfortable training pace allows you to practice trail skills without the stress of a steep grade. Be careful, however, when running downhill on sketchy sections of trail. For someone who is not used to running trails, the momentum gained from even a slight decline may result in a pace that is too quick for handling trail obstacles.

Once you become comfortable with both hills and trails, it is time to combine the two training approaches. Running uphill on technical trails requires a lot of strength, balance, conditioning, a sense of pace, proper form, and mental toughness. Chapter 3 addresses the development of these skills. A good uphill runner is also a runner who knows when to walk. There are times when walking is much more efficient and even faster than running, so don't get caught up in the common beginner's mistake of thinking that it is wrong to walk. Knowing when to walk and when to run uphill is a valuable asset that comes with experience.

Running downhill on trails is an acquired skill that draws on a runner's agility and confidence. A good descent requires quick feet, lateral stability, balance, and the ability to look beyond the next footstep so that you can prepare or "set up" for steps without having to slow forward progress as you are assisted by gravity.

SHOES

Those new to trail running often wonder whether they need to purchase new shoes for the sport. Although shoes designed specifically for running trails offer certain advantages over road-running shoes or light hiking or "approach" shoes, it is not necessary for someone who has comfortable road or lightweight cross-training shoes to invest in trail-specific running footwear prior to their first trail run.

Nonetheless, one may certainly enhance the initial trail running experience by wearing shoes that help rather than hinder the runner's ability to perform on uneven terrain at a running pace. This is especially true for the novice trail runner who has special needs due to foot or stride irregularities. Proper trail footwear is also important if you are likely to be on trails that require substantial traction, cushioning, or protection. While a road shoe may provide ample cushioning or support, it may lack in traction, provide inadequate protection from bone bruises, or wear too quickly, given the rigors of the trail. Conversely, a light hiking or approach shoe might offer plenty of traction, but it is likely to be too stiff and heavy for running.

Should you decide to purchase a pair of trail shoes, there are several important considerations that should go into the shopping decision. Although these considerations are addressed in detail in Chapter 7, as a first-time trail shoe buyer you will want to steer clear of paying top dollar for some gimmicky shoe. Given that you will not yet know what does and doesn't work for you on the trails, you should shoot for a more basic model of trail shoe (frequently called "entry-level") and one that is more of a hybrid shoe that functions well on both trail and road. If you are converting from road to trail and have a favorite brand of shoe for its fit and performance, it is a pretty safe bet that one of that company's trail shoes will be a suitable choice for a first trail shoe.

In selecting trail running footwear, consider personal characteristics such as susceptibility to particular foot or knee injuries or the need for additional support, stability, or motion control. Certain styles of trail shoes offer more support than others, and some help to correct stride idiosyncrasies. Thinking about the type of trails you will be on and their likely conditions will also help guide your initial trail shoe purchase. If the terrain is likely to be dry and rocky and the temperatures hot, then the proper shoe would vary dramatically from one that would be selected for wet, muddy, and cold conditions.

APPAREL AND EQUIPMENT

If you are coming to trail running from either a running or outdoors background, it is likely that you have the fundamental apparel and equipment for running trails. Trail running is not a high-fashion endeavor, and it is often pursued by those who wear the same gear they have had for years.

Proper attire for trail running is rather basic, revolving around the concept of layering garments to moderate body temperature, wick perspiration, and provide protection from the elements. Keep dry by minimizing or at least reducing sweat from inside and rain or snow from outside by following basic layering principles. The first layer—the layer closest to the skin—should be made of a comfortable, resilient material that pulls moisture from the skin where it can be transferred away from the body. Underwear, both briefs and bras, are also in the base layer category, and those garments should also wick moisture while providing an element of support.

The second layer is worn only when the conditions are such that warmth through insulation is necessary. A fleece vest is a common second layer. It serves to assist in the moisture transfer that started with the base layer and provides a lightweight method of maintaining warmth, especially when used in conjunction with an outer or third layer. Outerwear is indispensable when it comes to running trails during inclement weather. It protects against rain, sleet, snow, wind, etc. and should be breathable enough to allow perspiration to escape.

Don't forget to think about your head and hands. Almost any hat, cap, or other head covering will help protect against sun, excessive moisture loss, and exposure to the cold. Likewise, most mittens and gloves will be adequate for keeping the fingers warm, although mittens are invariably warmer than gloves. Sunglasses reduce or eliminate ultraviolet rays and glare, and also protect the eyes from airborne particles on windy days.

Finally, bring along water or a sports drink. Depending on the length of the planned trail run, it may be a good idea to carry some type of hydration system and to bring some food and a first-aid kit.

BASIC TIPS BEFORE HEADING OUT

1. Schedule a run with a friend or let someone know your planned route.
2. Carry a map when running in unfamiliar areas.
3. Drink plenty of water and take food or energy drinks for runs lasting more than one hour.
4. Dress for changing weather conditions.
5. Always be aware of your surroundings.

Whether you head for the trails alone or with a group, for competition, exercise, or a mental recharge, you will surely find enjoyment around every switchback.

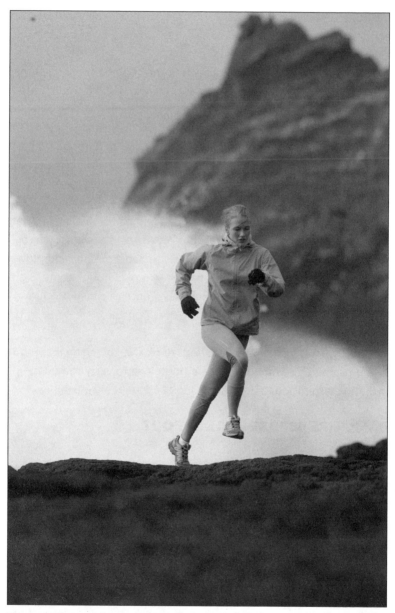

The power of your environment can motivate you like little else. Stephan/Gripmaster

CHAPTER 3

Trail Running Technique

Proper technique when running trails enables you to go faster and longer. Similarly, proper form allows you to run with less impact or stress and a decreased susceptibility to injury. If you are faster and healthier and have more stamina, then you are likely to be more motivated and approach running with greater confidence.

Running trails with a sense of purpose and strength is an invigorating experience that cultivates a deep sense of satisfaction, one that overflows into and supplements a fulfilling life. This chapter is about how to adopt proper technical form, which can lead to efficient and satisfying trail running.

ASCENTS

When observing the fastest and most efficient hill runners—both human and animal—it is easy to note their sustained turnover and shortened stride on the climb. Although their pace is slower on the ascent, such climbers manage to maintain a steady cadence.

The goal to running uphill on trails should be economy. The objective is to get to the top of the hill with the least amount of effort while maintaining a strong and steady pace. Different running styles work more efficiently for different runners, and the same runner may need to alternate between running, power hiking, charging, or even bounding up a hill, depending on the length, grade, and where the hill falls in a run. Fortunately, several universal techniques apply to trail ascents.

Shorten Your Stride

One piece of advice that three top mountain goat ultra trail runners—Jonathan Wyatt, Matt Carpenter, and Ian Torrence—offer for more efficient climbing is to "downshift" to a short stride using small but efficient steps. Kirk Apt, past winner of the Hardrock 100, one of the most difficult trail races in the world, compares running big ascents to riding a bike but recognizes that, unlike a bike, there is always another lower gear when you are on your feet. He says that it often helps him to repeat the mantra "rhythm, tempo, momentum, form" to maintain movement up a steep climb. But he tells runners to use anything that works to continue their grind up a hill. "Steady forward progress" is a common philosophy that applies to keeping up a pace to the spot where you can see the top of a climb, at which point, if you feel strong, you can pick up the cadence.

A shorter stride enables you to maintain a steady rhythm yet remain relatively light on your feet. With light feet, you are able to lift yourself over barriers and, when necessary, lunge to place your feet on top of solid footing in the trail. Climbing with more rapid steps also allows you to quickly alter direction and select the best route, one that offers the best traction and fewer obstacles. Depending on the amount of purchase you are able to maintain, given the trail surface and grade, you will want to strike your foot on either the toe first or the whole foot, positioning it to match the slope of the trail. Different foot strikes work better for different runners and under different circumstances, so experiment to find out which foot positions are most effective for you.

Avoid favoring one leg as the "power leg," a practice that is too frequently relied on for pushing off in order to drive up the hill. Instead, alternate using both legs for planting and pushing in order to remain equally balanced without developing disproportionate strength between the legs. Such balance enables a more even ascent and obviates the need to stutter step by taking off from the stronger leg in an effort to hurdle an approaching barrier on the trail.

Proper Form on the Ascent

Posture is an integral aspect of climbing because of its dual effect on breathing and the pressure or pain that ascending with bad posture can cause to the back. Try not to lean too far forward and resist the tendency to bend forward at the waist, as this will result in a sore lower back. When you feel the urge to lean forward, let your head and shoulders lean into the hill while keeping your mid and lower back straight. A straighter trunk allows for a fuller range of motion in the hip flexors and opens the breathing passage without compressing the digestive tract—which otherwise can lead to an upset stomach. An upright stance also improves traction and pushoff.

Concentrate on leg motion and take steady breaths to keep oxygen flowing to the back of the legs—glutes, hamstrings, and calves. Use the hip flexors to pick up the knees, and swing the arms with the same rapid rhythm as the legs. Use a steady arm swing to power up the hills and maintain forward momentum. Apt sometimes visualizes a rope being suspended from the top of the climb and pretends to grab it (without crossing his arms over his body) to pull himself up with each forward arm swing.

Keep your head up to facilitate looking up the trail to plan the next steps. Stay simultaneously focused on both present and near-future location as you ascend.

Walking Uphill

When you cannot maintain a consistent running pace or feel as though the effort to do so is overly exhausting, downshift and transition immediately into a fast walking pace or power hike. Depending on one's running style, the grade, footing, exhaustion level, and the altitude, power hiking may be more efficient and possibly even faster than running. The shift from a slow shuffle to a fast walk should be a smooth one initiated to keep the heart rate steady.

Individual runners develop their own style of power walking, depending on biomechanics and leg length. Some use a short, somewhat choppy gait with an erect posture that draws strength from the back of the legs. Others deploy long, almost lunging strides, leaning forward at the waist and relying on quadriceps. Some who use this latter technique, especially on steep grades, will actually place their hands on their knees to help push off with each step.

Torrence, a dominant trail ultramarathoner, recognizes that he can use power walking to climb some hills just as fast as he would if he were to run them. He recommends practicing on hills to test which grades are best for walking. "Running steep hills early at a high effort can leave you weak later in the run. Pace your hill climbing. Take them easier near the start of your run, then progressively increase effort as you close in on the finish."

Barriers, Obstacles, and Switchbacks

When confronted with rocks, fallen trees, water bars (the barriers that are placed to direct runoff to the side of the trail), and other obstacles that lay across the trail on mountain ascents, avoid stepping directly on the objects. Instead of wasting motion to lift your entire body weight straight up, time your steps to land as close to the barrier as possible so that the next step can easily clear the obstacle and land above it on the trail.

On steep, rocky, irregular terrain, runners with strong quads and long legs may find it best to deploy lengthy strides that drive up at least the first part of an ascent. When the lactic acid builds from such an effort, it may be necessary to slow for a moment until the burning of the muscles subsides before hitting it again. For those with weaker quads or shorter legs, a condensed stride is usually more efficient and effective.

When confronting switchbacks, you can eliminate unnecessary steps by pivoting on one foot, especially when the trail's surface is coated with loose gravel. It also is efficient to run the trail's tangents, hugging the curves as you climb.

Hill Running Recovery and Preparation

Uphill running taxes and strains rear leg muscles as well as hip flexors, quads, and the lower back. Accordingly, it is a good idea to stretch before and after hilly runs. Ice, cold water, and/or massage may also be a good idea.

What if you do not live near any hills? Find a local stadium or skyscraper and do repeats on the stairs, but be careful of footing. Alternatively, go to a gym and use a stair-climbing machine or treadmill with a steep-grade setting. Another option is to use a spinning bike set on high tension. You can simulate "running" on the pedals by standing above the saddle. Yet there is no real substitute for climbing preparation other than actually hitting the hills.

Hill Climbing
and Mental Magnets

By Roch Horton, ultra trail runner and fast packer from Salt Lake City, Utah

Many runners new to trail running are often stymied by the mere thought of actually running up steep trails for extended periods. Hiking up is tough enough, let alone running.

Like many other elements of off-road running, it all boils down to training. Whether it be stair climbing, hill repeats, weight machines, or even dragging an old tire around behind you as you run up dirt roads or ski hills, it all adds to strength and maneuverability on the run up.

Often overlooked, however, is the mental part of climbing hills. It is probably the rare trail runner who could recall their thoughts while grinding up a steep grade or endless switchbacks other than "this sucks" or "when's it end?" Here's an effective albeit silly tidbit I resort to when I feel the pull of gravity taking its toll on those long hills.

First I visualize a giant magnet mounted at a specific destination. This could be at the top of a high pass or the next aid station in a race. It's a giant magnet, painted bright red, complete with little magnetic lightning bolts coming out of it, like something you would see in an old *Jetsons* cartoon. It's pointed right at me. Embedded in my chest is a weightless steel plate. I control the size of the plate. Negative thoughts or whining . . . it gets smaller. Positive thoughts, eating or drinking something, relaxed breathing, standing tall, looking around . . . it grows larger; and as a result the more pull I can feel coming from the magnet. By aiming my way up the trail toward the magnet, the climb gets just a bit easier. Remember, that magnet can't replace the aforementioned training. And remember also to disengage the magnet when you head down the other side!

DESCENTS

Bob Dion, a fixture in the New England trail racing scene, is known for his ability to make up time on his competition by attacking descents at breakneck speed. Skilled downhill runners can use their ability to descend steep trails and overtake unskilled downhill runners who struggle with exertion from the ascent. In a long run with many hills, energy conservation is crucial. Because it takes less effort to run downhill quickly than to climb at a rapid pace, talented downhill runners finish runs more rested than those who are less skilled at trail descents.

Proper Form on the Descent

When running downhill, avoid the tendency to lean back in an effort to slow down or to lean too far forward and overstride. Body weight should be centered over the knees with each foot striking on the ball rather than heel. This will prevent you from leaning back, which is inefficient and can lead to back pain and knee damage. Maintain a relaxed pose, with your elbows slightly raised and some levity in your arms. When making a sharp turn or maneuvering a steep dropoff during a descent, lift your arms and shoulders a bit higher to help maintain balance and shock absorption thanks to a loaded spring effect. This posture gives you a slightly aggressive forward or downhill lean and a faster descent, so be wary, because the pace may be more rapid and challenging than you are used to handling.

Perfect your downhill running form a little at a time, especially if you are new to running quickly downhill or when descending on trails with tricky footing. To learn proper trail descending technique, start by running down smooth, gradual hills before progressing by adding steepness and technical footing, preferably one at a time.

Look Ahead

The key to quick descents is looking beyond your feet—something that mountain bikers and mogul and Alpine skiers can appreciate. Focus on the bigger picture and less on nearby details. Merely scan upcoming trail and terrain features rather than getting bogged down with the specific placement of every step.

Trail running is like skiing the trees. You've got to focus on seeing those smooth spaces between the rocks and obstacles.
—Jeannie Wall, accomplished trail runner, mountain climber, and backcountry and Nordic skier who resides in Bozeman, Montana

Good trail descenders need to "be" ahead of where they actually are. This may sound like Chevy Chase in *Caddyshack* talking about "being" the ball, but the objective is to anticipate, like a chess player who mentally projects and develops moves for a winning strategy. By looking ahead, you can "set up" for turns or finesse large obstacles by shifting your weight, adjusting your gait, timing your steps, and avoiding sudden changes in direction or speed.

Quiet the Feet and Shorten the Stride

Your feet should be relatively quiet on the trail, even when descending. The sound of your feet thundering down the trail pounding out each step is likely to translate to sore back and quadriceps pain, and possible knee injury. Maintain a steady rhythm without sacrificing flexibility in cadence. Remember, it is far better to jump over fallen trees, unsteady rocks, or other obstacles than to step on them.

Employing many little steps facilitates making minor directional adjustments and controlling speed. Increasing the number of steps you take is an efficient way to govern descent pace and prevent joint and impact injuries. It is like putting a car in a lower gear instead of riding the brakes when driving a steep decline. By increasing foot turnover, you will decrease the impulse to lean backward and attempt to brake with the heels, which causes stress to the hamstrings and tendons. This frequent-step technique also allows you to maintain some spring in your step because you will keep your knees slightly bent without locking or hyperextending. To help you stay light on your feet, focus on speed, aggressiveness, and confidence during descents.

Maintain a Float

Good downhill trail runners have mastered the ability to run technical downhill sections at a fast pace and maintain a "float" over varying terrain. A float occurs when runners keep a smooth and steady upper body while their legs and trunk move laterally and pivot backward and forward to maneuver the descent. By perfecting that float, trail runners can save an incredible amount of energy while running faster descents.

Maintaining a fluid, observant composure when descending trails will help you relax. With proper running form and a honed sense of proprioception, you will be better able to maneuver the best route down the trail. This may be difficult to do if you are injured or fearful from prior falls, so slow your pace until you gain the confidence that translates into relaxation. Breathe steadily, resist the impulse to tense up, and avoid sudden or jerky movements.

Man is born gentle and supple.
At death, his body is brittle and hard.
...
The stiff, the hard, the brittle are harbingers of death,
and gentleness and yielding are signs of that which lives.
The warrior who is inflexible condemns himself to death,
and the tree is easily broken, which ever refuses to yield.
Thus the hard and brittle will surely fall, and the soft and supple
will overcome.

—Lao-tzu, *Tao Te Ching*

Lisa Jhung, a trail runner from Boulder, Colorado, also subscribes to the importance of running relaxed on descents. She recommends letting go, loosening up the shoulders, kicking up the heels, flopping the arms as though swimming through the air, and flowing freely, allowing you to enjoy the momentum of the downhill. "Running free and floppy downhill is better on joints and muscles because you're not trying to overcontrol and restrain every motion."

Cornering

To ease the descent, remember that even though the shortest distance between two points is a straight line, it is often more graceful to maintain speed by approaching and coming out of curves in wide angles. Like

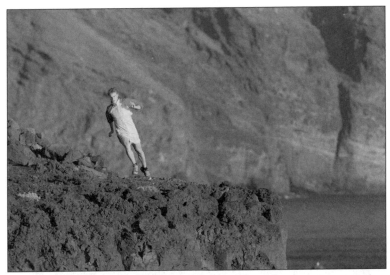

Maintaining balance as you accelerate through turns can be exhilarating. Stephan/Gripmaster

bike racers going into a corner, when you are running trails you can go at almost full speed by entering and exiting at broad tangents and cutting as close as possible to the inside of the turn. This technique permits you to hold a steady, quick clip on the descent.

Falling Technique

Competitive mogul skiers train to follow a straight route called a "fall line." You should do the same to reduce lateral motion and take the most efficient route down the trail. Unfortunately, the term "fall line" is also apropos to trail running because trail runners occasionally lose their balance and have more contact with the earth than they would prefer.

Falling is an unfortunate inevitability of downhill trail running. Knowing how best to fall with minimal damage is a skill that is learned in the school of hard knocks. Depending on what triggers the fall—catching a toe on a root, slipping on loose rock or ice, or merely being a klutz—you may be able to recover before you hit the ground by redistributing weight if you respond in time. A long stride or lateral "catch" may be enough to steady the body, but sometimes such corrective attempts are not worth it because they can cause muscle strain, joint damage, or throw the body's weight off in the other direction.

Dave Mackey, a downhill speedster, rarely falls when he descends, but he advises those who do fall to "stop, drop, and roll" (except on rocky, cactus-laden, or treed terrain). He cautions against the urge to put your hands out to stop the fall because that can lead to broken wrists. Mackey also recommends that, even when falling, you should remain relaxed and flexible.

Your goal should always be to emerge from a fall without any serious injury. To do this, absorb a fall with the greatest available amount of soft tissue and body mass while protecting your head. Rolling or sliding is usually the best bet, especially if the alternative is a twisted or torqued ankle, knee, or elbow. To develop falling skills, find a grassy hill, put on layers of old sweats for padding, and practice rolling and sliding. If prone to ankle problems, wear higher-collared shoes, wrap ankles, or investigate another kind of ankle support.

Feel the Burn?

By toning muscles through consistent downhill training you will be able to reduce the burning feeling that is caused by the buildup of the chemical creatine phosphokinase (CPK), which is produced by muscles while descending. The pain from CPK is similar to the burning feeling caused by a buildup of lactic acid, and can last for days. Running in a relaxed, flowing style will help to minimize CPK buildup.

TERRAIN

More than anything else, varying terrain distinguishes trail running from road running. The challenge and excitement of confronting mud, snow, ice, water crossings, roots, rocks, and other obstacles of the trail keeps trail running dynamic and forces us to be ever vigilant about maintaining a broad base of trail running skills. The following sections discuss particular techniques for dealing with specific types of terrain that you are likely to encounter on the trails.

Mud

The best way to deal with mud on the trail is to enjoy it and to get as dirty as possible early in the run so you won't worry about it thereafter. Soft mud enables a lower-impact run. On descents, it provides a great surface for slowing the pace without stressing joints.

Mud and Footwear

If you know the trail will be muddy, wear older shoes that still have secure collars around the ankles to prevent or limit mud seepage into the shoes. Make sure your shoes are securely fastened so they do not end up being sucked right off in deep mud. Losing a shoe in deep mud is a humbling experience—you will end up kneeling sock-footed with your arm submerged in deep muck trying to fish out a shoe that the trail has seemingly devoured.

Mud and Body Positioning

To avoid slipping, it may help to shorten your stride, run more upright than normal, and keep your elbows angled and slightly elevated for lateral balance. This posture centers your gravity and allows you to react quickly in the event that your feet lose traction. If you begin to slip, try to relax and control the recovery so as not to overreact and fall in the opposite direction.

With the well-deserved nickname of "Mud 'N Guts," Dana Miller's general advice for trail runners confronting mud is to "slow down a bit, try to run more relaxed so you can recover from a slip better, and choose your footing more carefully." Miller cautions against attempting to try to stay clean and dry: "Hey, this is trail running! Get dirty, have fun, be a kid again!"

Know Your Mud

If water is running down a trail creating a muddy slope, your best bet is to run where water is moving most rapidly (usually the center of the trail) because that will probably be the most firm. A faster current tends to remove most of the sticky sediment, leaving behind gravel and rock. Although you will get a little wet, the likelihood of getting bogged down by sticky mud is markedly decreased. This technique is also friendlier to the trail as it has less of an environmental impact.

If you have some familiarity with the area and its soil makeup, then you can discern the content of the mud from its color and texture. Shiny mud usually has higher water content, which may mean it is more slippery, and if it is deep it could have greater suction power—like quicksand. If the mud has high clay content, count on running with heavy feet through the muddy section of the trail. Once through the clay, either scrape the mud off your feet or find a body of water for a cleansing splash and dash.

From an environmental standpoint, resist the temptation to run alongside the trail in an effort to avoid getting muddy. This practice leads to wider trails; and if everyone did it, pathways would soon be major throughways instead of singletrack trails. Depending on the sensitivity of the region's trail system, it may be advisable to avoid certain trails during typically muddy times of the year.

Snow and Ice

Running with confidence is more important on snow and ice than on any other surface. Most runners are hesitant on snow and ice, but the trick is to try to tuck away that insecurity, take a deep breath, and run with a sense of command. Although snow and ice—being inanimate elements—cannot read minds, they somehow manage to wreak havoc on runners who fear them. Fearful runners run with tense form, lean back, and often resort to jerky, sudden movements in an attempt to adapt to the slick surface. That is just the opposite of what works best.

The best form for snow and ice running is a slight forward lean that distributes the body's weight evenly across the foot as it hits the slippery surface. Fluid, steady movement is less likely to cause a loss of traction. In the event of slipping on snow or ice, the best response is to relax and to try to let your body flow with a calculated response. Resist the impulse to tense up or make a sudden movement to counter the slipping, which all too often leads to slipping even more or injury.

Many trail runners use snowshoes when running in the winter as a way to keep up trail running fitness. Running on snowshoes during the winter snowpack allows you to stay on the same trails year-round. The snow's forgiving compressibility and the absorption from snowshoes' increased surface area are also attractive qualities to winter snowshoe running.

Water Crossings

Do you recall running through large puddles—or even small ponds—as a child? If so, then you probably mastered the technique of taking exaggerated giant steps that kept you relatively dry while making everyone near you wet. That same technique is invaluable to trail running, and if you don't have it down, take advantage of the dampness and warmth during spring to hone it. Go to a shallow stream, puddle, or other body of water that is not more than 6 inches deep. When crossing large, shallow puddles, use an extended, high-stepping stride, and throw a little lateral kick and flourish at the end of each step to push the water away.

Deep Water Crossings

For deeper water crossings, decide whether it is worth trying to stay dry. The water and air temperature, the width of the body of water, the rate of the current, the availability of an alternative, and the amount of time you can afford should factor into your decision. Many people have been carried to their deaths by fast-moving currents, so make sure that you will be able to safely navigate the crossing.

Scout possible crossings and avoid charging into streams and rivers only to find logs and rocks that would have allowed for dry, safe passage. Likewise, do not get too excited about jumping into the water if the stream or riverbed contains large jagged rocks. Seek a shallow place to cross or do some boulder hopping. If you are feeling fatigued, you will have a difficult time maintaining your balance, so exercise some real caution. When making water crossings, watch for deep holes, and if the water is expected to be above knee level or is running with a strong current, use a stick or link arms with a running mate or two to help maintain balance and forward momentum.

Water Crossings and Footwear

Though using waterproof breathable shoes or carrying a change of socks can help, there is no foolproof method for keeping your feet dry. As an alternative, consider the "easy in/easy out" approach of wearing highly breathable shoes with mesh uppers. This allows water to penetrate the foot when confronting water crossings, but they also allow water to exit quickly. Water will be effectively squeegeed out of your shoes by running on dry terrain, and after a mile or two the recent drenching will be only a faint memory. Wearing wool socks, especially ones made with merino wool, which does not itch, will maintain a moderate temperature for your feet regardless of whether they are wet or dry. They will also help prevent blisters and ward off odor with their natural antimicrobial attributes.

Dana Miller takes a somewhat religious approach to water crossings: "If you're talking about the Red Sea, Moses is the expert. Trust God and let him do the work. It's kind of like that in trail running . . . the water's not going to hurt you, but those rocks underneath might."

ROOTS, ROCKS, FALLEN BRANCHES, AND OTHER TRAIL OBSTACLES

In *Daniels' Running Formula*, Jack Daniels explains why those who run on rougher terrain need not run too quickly: "There are those runners whose environment may be mostly slow footing, such as sand, grass, gravel roads, and rocky trails. . . . Residents of slow-footing environments learn to be strength runners and also develop good resistance to many injuries because they are constantly dealing with twisting and turning feet."

Obstacle Avoidance

When running on a particularly difficult section of trail, it is often beneficial to lift your knees a little higher than usual. This, in turn, will pick your feet up a little higher off the ground, giving more clearance to avoid catching a toe or otherwise tripping on a rock, root, or other potential snag. Use the forward vision technique previously discussed with respect to trail descents; this helps you select a relatively clear line in the trail that, in turn, will help you to maintain speed without losing balance or twisting an ankle.

Depending on your running style, the length of your run, and the distance traveled, you may find it easiest to use a shorter stride and to run through rough footing with lighter but more rapid steps. Running on your toes, the way football players—hardly known for their daintiness—run through tire obstacle courses, takes weight off your feet so that you can quickly adjust your balance and recover from any misstep. Of course, this is difficult to do when you are tired and your legs and feet feel heavy and sluggish.

You may be frequently confronted with the dilemma of whether it is best to jump over, go around, or step on top of a fallen tree, branch, rock, or other obstacle. Even though the decision to jump or not is driven by numerous factors, you must make the decision instantaneously. Some of the more substantial variables in the equation are the speed at which you approach the obstacle, the size and stability of the obstacle, your general agility and experience, the footing leading to and from the obstacle, and your general level of chutzpah or cunning.

Once you have made the lightning-fast decision of whether to go over or around an obstacle, embrace the decision with confidence and leap over, step on, or steer around the barrier without second-guessing yourself. Do not dwell on a botched decision, but learn from mistakes so as to be better able to tackle the next trail barrier. The element of surprise, the challenge of uncertainty, and the never-ending supply of varying obstacles are what make trail running exciting. If these uncertainties do not make for fun and excitement, then run roads.

Trail races celebrate the wild side of running. . . strength, agility, and toughness reign here, rather than pure speed. Entry forms brag about the difficulties of the course, and finishers proudly emerge from the woods mud splattered, scraped, torn, and bleeding (bleeding is not mandatory but certainly not discouraged). Times and distances mean far less in this world than on the roads, and runners rarely settle into a steady pace or rhythm.

—Jonathan Beverly, "Preparing for Your Race Distance"
in *Breakthrough Running*

Mental Focus

Tim Twietmeyer, five-time winner of the Western States 100, observes that "varying trail conditions and scenery provide a constant mental challenge, whether it's avoiding rocks on the trail, reading the course markings, or taking in the views from the hilltops." Trail running takes a lot of mental focus because of the constant need to anticipate and deal with obstacles. Whether it is roots, rocks, branches, logs, bushes, or animal droppings, you will constantly be barraged, and if you want to run at a quick clip and avoid falling, then you should be prepared to miss some of the scenery.

ALTITUDE

The statement that high-altitude trails are breathtaking has two meanings. Beauty above timberline is outstanding. One may revel in the pristine clarity of glacier lilies, bluebells, and scarlet paintbrush while chuckling to the humor of pika chirps. Best of all, the uninhibited views from what feels like the top of the world are awe inspiring.

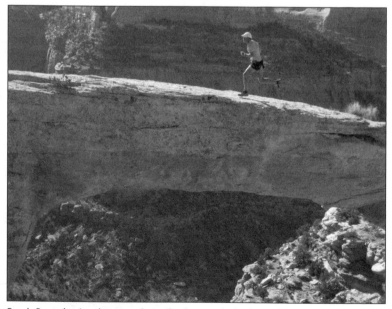

Bernie Boettcher is at home on the trails, always enjoying beautiful locations and seeking adventure. Bernie Boettcher

To earn those views, however, you must come to grips with the reality that running at higher elevations is physically demanding. You should also acknowledge the risks that accompany high-altitude running, especially if you are running at a high elevation without first acclimatizing from sea level. This section provides some explanation of the challenge of running trails at altitude, including a discussion of heart rate and its monitoring.

Effects of Altitude on Performance

Exertion at higher altitudes is more difficult than at sea level because of the reduced partial pressure of oxygen as elevation rises. The decrease in oxygen pressure impairs the oxygenation of blood flowing through the lungs, which ultimately results in a corresponding diminished oxygen supply to working muscles. Studies by the Federation of Sport at Altitude have shown that the lack of oxygen at elevations above 10,000 feet translates to 25 to 40 percent less muscle power (depending on the individual). At 16,400 feet above sea level, partial oxygen pressure is approximately half of that at sea level. Trail runners should acclimatize by training at an altitude of about 8,000 feet for at least four or five days before running above 13,000 feet, although such acclimatization is not required for runners who live above 6,500 feet.

The human body requires a constant supply of oxygen from ambient air to maintain the process of aerobic metabolism. Even though the percentage of oxygen in the air remains constant regardless of altitude, the decrease in pressure relative to an increase in altitude translates into a diminished oxygen-hemoglobin association. In short, the higher the altitude, the less the amount of oxygen carried in the bloodstream.

Physiological Adaptation to Altitude

To compensate for the reduced oxygen delivery to the bloodstream at altitude, the heart must work harder and faster to maintain the same absolute performance or pace. The heart compensates for the diminution of oxygen through an increase in cardiac output, or the amount of blood pumped by each heartbeat.

Blood composition is another way the body compensates for altitude. After approximately fourteen to sixty days of altitude acclimatization, the body produces more red blood cells and hemoglobin—the iron-protein compound that transports oxygen. Altitude also causes the kidneys to increase production of erythropoietin or EPO, which stimulates bone marrow production to increase both the concentration of red cells in the blood and total plasma volume. This explains why EPO has been a favorite substance for drug-doping endurance competitors who try to find a shortcut to greater fitness. An additional adaptation to altitude is that working muscle tissue learns to rely on more fatty acids, rather than the common glycogen source of energy fuel. These gradual adaptations result in a reduction of the cardiac output required for oxygen delivery during exercise.

The virtues of altitude training for endurance athletes have been touted since the 1968 Olympic Games in Mexico City, situated at 7,349 feet, where it was established that performance at high altitude demands training at high altitude. Studies have shown, however, that the physiological response to altitude training varies widely, depending upon individual characteristics. Accordingly, the following discussion of trail running at altitude is general in nature, and you should consider the advice of a qualified coach, exercise physiologist, health care professional, or other certified trainer in individualizing your altitude training or racing.

Monitoring of Resting Heart Rate

Understanding the association of heart rate and altitude will help you to appreciate the effects of altitude. Fundamental to that understanding, you should be familiar with the monitoring of your heart. Cardiac output—the amount of blood pumped per minute—is a function of heart rate and stroke volume (the amount of blood pumped by each heartbeat). Your resting heart rate is often used as the baseline against which to measure your heart rate during exercise. While resting heart rates vary from individual to individual, they offer a good measure of baseline fitness, which in turn can be an indicator of overtraining when the same person tracks his or her rate from day to day. Resting heart rate is usually measured first thing in the morning. You can do this when you are in a relaxed state by manually taking your pulse for a timed interval.

Place your index and middle fingers on your neck, on the right side of your throat, and count the number of beats for a twenty-second period. Multiply that number by three to get the number of beats per minute, which is your resting heart rate. Alternatively, you can measure your heart rate by simply attaching a heart rate monitor and relaxing for a few minutes in a seated or reclined position so that you allow your rate to drop to its lowest level. Monitored on a daily or weekly basis, a trend toward slower heart rate often indicates improved fitness, while a trend toward higher rates may indicate overtraining, dehydration, nutritional deficiencies, illness, or increased stress.

Monitoring of Exercising Heart Rate

Monitoring heart rate during exercise provides a measure of the intensity of the workout. Increased intensity corresponds to higher heart rate, assuming that all things are equal, because there is a linear relationship between heart rate, workload, and oxygen consumption. With improved fitness, an individual may increase the intensity of exercise while maintaining the same or even lowered heart rate.

Each individual's general or background heart rate is unique, but certain variations are attributable to sex, age, overall health and fitness, size, sleep patterns, and lifestyle. Given one's background heart rate, individual factors such as temperature, clothing, hydration, diet, terrain, type of exercise and body position, humidity, stress, altitude, time of day, and a variety of other influences have an impact on a person's specific heart rate. These variations should be accounted for when comparing your heart rate from day to day and may explain what would otherwise be unexplainable changes.

Nonetheless, by monitoring your heart rate on a regular basis you will be able to gauge your general effort and avoid overtraining by controlling workout intensity, especially under conditions where it would otherwise be difficult to accurately measure your pace—such as running on undulating trails with a multitude of obstacles. Matt Carpenter, a champion performer at high-altitude mountain running (who is known as "lungs on legs"), compares heart rate monitoring to driving an automobile with an instrument panel. The monitor allows you to gauge your body for signs of trouble or, more hopefully, signs of progress. A pulse monitor can become an indispensable training partner that gives instant feedback and a sense of control and direction during workouts.

The goal of endurance athletes is to be able to perform as close as possible to maximum oxygen consumption—known as "VO_2 max"—without suffering from a high accumulation of lactic acid. Lactic acid is produced as a by-product of working muscles. When the concentration of lactic acid rises too high, the result is a burning sensation, pain, muscle fatigue, and cramping or seizing. The point where blood-lactate concentrations become too high to further increase the workload or pace is measured as a percentage of one's VO_2 max. That measure is known as either the lactate or anaerobic threshold.

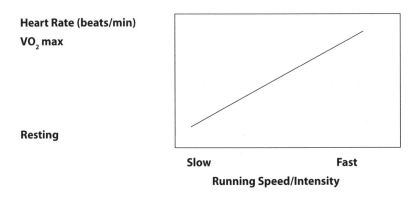

Each person's lactate threshold is unique and changes with age. At exertion levels below the lactate threshold, oxygen remains the primary source of energy. However, when intensity is increased to an anaerobic level, such as during a sprint, the body draws on stored sugars or glycogen for energy. The point where the body converts from using oxygen to glycogen demarks your lactate threshold. Proper training will raise a person's lactate threshold so that it corresponds to a higher percentage of VO_2 max.

Effect of Altitude on Heart Rate

The effects of altitude on the heart generally begin at approximately 3,048 feet (1,000 meters) above sea level. The decrease in oxygen delivered to working muscles translates into a decrease in VO_2 max at altitude. Maintaining the same level of intensity experienced at sea level requires a decrease in pace when at altitude. Consequently, athletes who do all of their training at altitude may sacrifice quality training because they are unable to achieve the kind of leg speed or turnover they experience with the same effort at sea level. To compensate for the slower pace at altitude and work on leg speed, some runners who live at altitude do some speed drills on a slight decline or ride stationary bikes at a high cadence.

Although the slower pace of interval and threshold training at altitude translates to faster relative speed at sea level, experts debate the value of the fitness benefits relative to the decreased ability to train hard at altitude. The growing consensus is that it is ideal to "live high and train low" to get the best of both worlds. Some athletes who live at lower elevations have taken this principle to mean sleep high and train low and have equipped their bedrooms or sleep chambers with devices that convert the barometric pressure from 6,000 feet to as high as 16,000 feet to achieve some of the physiological benefits of high altitude.

If you are training at altitude with the goal of performing well at sea level, your altitude workout pace should equal or approach your sea-level goal pace. To achieve that objective may require taking longer recoveries during workouts or using shorter interval distances.

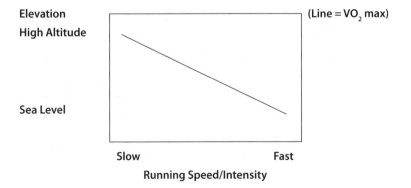

Elevation
High Altitude

Sea Level

(Line = VO_2 max)

Slow   Fast

Running Speed/Intensity

Performance improvements gained from altitude training are relatively long lasting, as is one's overall level of fitness. Athletes who train at altitude have obtained breakthroughs in their performance and reached goals they had been unable to achieve with sea-level training. Altitude training has been compared to high-mileage or interval training. Moreover, the increased stress of altitude on the body, especially during athletic competition, has lasting physiological effects.

Dangers of Running at Altitude

You should be aware of other altitude factors that can affect your heart rate, such as length of your acclimatization at altitude, highest altitude attained, intensity of the climb, ascent rate, previous altitude experience, time at altitude, and the difficulty of the trail run, including the lack of traction.

When exercising at altitude, be alert to preliminary danger signs of dehydration, shortness of breath, lightheadedness, sore muscles, rapid heart rate, or headaches. Drink more at altitude and allow for plenty of rest, including naps, if possible. Also be aware of increased cold, wind chill, exposure, intensity of UV rays from the sun, and possible sleep problems. All of these factors will affect your heart rate and general welfare.

Acute mountain sickness (AMS) plagues those who ascend too quickly, and it is most common among people who arrive at altitude from sea level without any period for acclimating. The acclimatization period will depend on a variety of factors, including the person's home base altitude, the destination altitude, fitness level, age, and past experiences at altitude. Symptoms of AMS include headaches, fatigue, irritability, constipation, disturbed sleep, loss of appetite, nausea, vomiting, flatulence, and a decrease in urine output despite proper hydration. These make for a debilitating combination that usually kicks in six to twelve hours after ascending to the higher elevation. AMS becomes most intense after a full day or two at altitude and takes as long as a week to dissipate through acclimatization.

AMS can be treated by descending, taking acetazolamide (Diamox) or dexamethasone, or through the use of a Gamow chamber, a device that effectively lowers the barometric pressure inside a pump-operated bivouac sack-type contraption. Some people are allergic to Diamox, while others suffer the side effect of frequent urination. Recent studies indicate that consumption of supplements of the herb ginkgo biloba may have a positive effect of limiting AMS, especially on slower ascents.

High-altitude cerebral edema (HACE) is an extreme case of AMS where the brain swells enough to cause loss of consciousness, but it also manifests itself through extreme fatigue and weakness, confusion, impaired mental faculties, staggered gait, loss of coordination, drowsiness, or even coma. HACE, which can be fatal, normally takes three days to develop, beginning as AMS. It can be treated the same way as AMS is remedied, but the sufferer should descend, take the same medications used for AMS, and consume supplemental oxygen.

A third high-altitude malady is high-altitude pulmonary edema (HAPE), which evidences itself through the symptoms of breathlessness, bluish skin, a hacking cough that produces a pink froth, rapid heart rate, and a clicking sound from the heart, called rales, that is caused by mucus buildup in the lungs, which can be detected through a stethoscope. AMS often accompanies HAPE. If untreated, HAPE can be fatal within twelve hours. To counteract HAPE, sufferers are given supplemental oxygen and plenty of rest or, if more severe, brought down from altitude and given the same medications used for AMS and HACE.

Trail Running at Altitude

Trail runners frequently train and race at altitude, where many standard rules of lowland running no longer apply. Marino Giacometti, president of the International Skyrunning Federation, observes that "running at high altitude forces you to adopt quite a different style from the normal rhythmic, consistent pace of low altitude." Although trail running at any altitude requires precision footwork, high-altitude runners must get used to the lack of a regular gait cycle because of uneven terrain and snow. High-altitude trail running frequently requires alternating running and walking, especially on steep inclines.

For those new to high-altitude running, it is best to adapt by focusing on maintaining a steady rhythm with regular breathing. Slow down and shorten your stride to keep from getting out of breath. Walk when necessary, especially when the grade exceeds 25 percent.

Joe Kulak, aka "Puking Joe," has a knack for vomiting during his ultras. He shares this with us:

> It was the night before the 2003 Leadville Trail 100 and I was busy making my last-minute plans. This would be my seventh Leadville in a row and the fourth 100-miler in the 2003 Last Great Race Series. With Old Dominion 100, Western States 100, and Vermont 100 behind me, I was anxious to grind out another Leadville.
>
> In typical fashion I drove up to Leadville with friends on Thursday night to be fresh for the race check-in Friday morning. My wife Kristen would drive up from Denver after work on Friday to join us for dinner. Well, 6:00 p.m. rolled around and all the runners were knee deep into the pasta feed when Kristen pulled into the dirt driveway. I went outside to meet her and she greeted me with a huge smile. She reached into her pocket and pulled out a pregnancy test stick revealing that she was pregnant. We embraced each other there on a little dirt driveway in Leadville, ecstatic that in nine months we would be parents of our first child. Throughout the next day the miles came and went, the skies opened up, and the vistas were beautiful. All along I was glowing in our newfound role as soon-to-be-parents. As morning sickness hit Kristen hard during the following weeks, we puked our way through the Wasatch Front 100 and Angeles Crest 100 and completed the Last Great Race eager to start our next journey. . . .

Ski Poles for High-Altitude Ascents

On high-altitude ascents, especially on rugged terrain or snow, some trail runners opt to use lightweight Nordic ski poles. Ski poles help distribute weight more evenly when ascending. This is key in high-altitude climbs because it promotes better blood circulation to the brain, thereby reducing hypoxia—the affliction that severely attacks nervous tissue. If you plan on using poles, practice climbing with them and learn to grip them properly. Perfect the technique and timing of planting them on the opposite side of the leading foot in a style similar to that of classical cross-country skiers. When running with ski poles on the flats or descents, carry them horizontally, both in one hand, to minimize their cumbersome qualities and keep them from getting in the way.

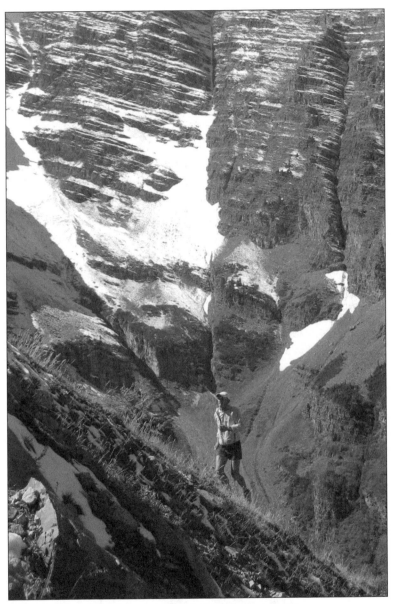

Bernie Boettcher enjoys mountain training in Colorado. Bernie Boettcher

Orientation at Altitude

Running above timberline requires that you are well oriented. It demands navigational skills due to the lack of trodden paths, signposts, or other directional landmarks. Combine that with a lack of oxygen to the brain and the concomitant disorientation of hypoxia, and it is easy to understand how you can get lost at high altitude or descend into an unintended drainage area and end up miles off course.

ULTRADISTANCE

The best way to train for long races is to do long training runs. When heading out for a long run, know the route and the trail conditions, anticipate the weather, and carry more than is necessary for a shorter run on the trails. Bring clothes to keep warm or cool, a map, and perhaps a cell phone. A crucial aspect of ultradistance training is to carry enough water and electrolytes to stay hydrated between water sources. If the route is without potable water sources, carry iodine tablets or a filter. To ward off cramps, bring an electrolyte replacement mix or mineral capsules. It is a good idea to do your long runs with a training partner. However, when doing a long run solo, make sure to inform someone of your planned route and then stick to it.

When racing an ultradistance trail event, make sure that you are familiar with the food and drink that will be available at the aid stations on the course. If the items offered don't work for you, take advantage of drop bag opportunities and strategically place your own special fuels along the course. Know the distance between aid stations and be sure to consume enough and/or carry enough to get from station to station.

In all ultras, finishing the distance is the primary goal of those who enter. "Go as you please" still describes the ultra pace—although some please to go remarkably fast. . . . Physical and mental endurance distinguish successful ultrarunners, who tend to keep their own company and eschew mainstream trends in clothing, training, and nutrition.

—Jonathan Beverly in "Preparing for Your Race Distance"
in *Breakthrough Running*

The two factors that distinguish ultra trail running from running shorter distances are pace and the ability to consume and use calories and liquids on the run. Most ultra DNFs (did not finishes) can ultimately be attributed to improper pacing or the failure to stay hydrated or fueled. Proper pacing and mastering the intake of drink and food is a real skill, which explains why successful ultradistance trail runners have both of those dialed.

Pace

One of the most common mistakes of a first-time ultrarunner is to go out too fast. Veteran ultrarunners know how to stay within their ability level and maintain a steady, almost metronomic, pace. Kirk Apt, past winner of the Hardrock 100, is known for his "slow and steady wins the race" approach to ultras. Apt is one of the only runners who is likely to run the second half of an ultra faster than the first. That "negative split" is almost unheard of because so many runners feel good at the beginning and want to make hay while the sun shines.

Ian Torrence, who won more trail ultramarathons in the first several years of the new millennium than any other runner in the same period, recognizes that it is easy to be sucked into another person's pace or become lost in the surrounding beauty. Resist both urges, because running too fast or losing focus early on in an ultra depletes your energy reserves, and that will come back to haunt you later in the run. Pacing does not, however, mean that you should run too slowly. Too slow a pace can lead to problems such as improper running form, which can cause connective tissue injury and force you to either miss a cutoff in an ultrarace, be pulled from the course, or run in the dark, the latter of which may be unavoidable but can at least be minimized.

In some of the longer or more challenging ultradistance trail events, the entire field will walk a portion of the course. Races such as the Hardrock 100 or the Barkley have been won at paces that are slower than eighteen minutes per mile, although those days are likely over now that the sport has been pushed to new, much-faster levels. Ultrarunners use walking to break up long steep ascents, and often use some power walking. Walking allows ultrarunners to refuel, give some running muscles a break, and relax the mind without actually stopping progress toward the goal of finishing. Tim Twietmeyer, finisher of more than eighty ultras, recommends practicing walking. In his first 50-miler, he walked a portion of every ten-minute section of the race. "I was pretty wasted at the end, but I was still able to break seven hours. It's a lot more fun to feel like running portions of the entire distance than to run the first 70 percent and walk the last 30 percent."

Buzz Burrell and Peter Bakwin, who at one time held records on the Colorado Trail and the John Muir Trail for multiday trail running, adhere to the importance of pace by pushing to keep up their progress even when they are utterly exhausted. When running at high altitudes with blisters, fatigue, darkness, and extreme weather, Burrell and Bakwin kick into what is known as "RFM" mode: relentless forward motion. For such extreme endurance efforts, both have found that it is better to keep continuously on the move than to stop and go in spurts.

Stay Fueled

Beyond pace, ultrarunners must contend with the challenge of maintaining the body's delicate balance of hydration along with temperature regulation, minerals to prevent cramping, and fuel for brain and muscle function. Eat and drink early and often. Ultraruns are no time to diet or neglect nutritional intake. Doing so leads to problems such as "bonking," or running out of energy, stomach problems, or electrolyte imbalances. Failure to take in liquids, salts, and fuel leave ultrarunners depleted—a deficit from which one does not easily recover. See Chapter 8 for more information on nutrition.

Mental and Emotional Challenges

While training and physical conditioning are absolutely crucial to ultradistance trail running, never underestimate the importance of the mental and emotional challenge confronting an ultrarunner. The trail demons that haunt ultradistance runs pervasively torture the soul while one is at the weakest moment in a race. Training will only get you so far; if you are not determined, focused, and goal oriented, the distance is likely to be your undoing. Those setting out to finish an ultra will go through bad times, may feel sick, will probably want to stop, and will probably swear they will never do one again . . . until about five minutes after they finish, when they will start planning their next event. Of course, not every runner suffers from such downs during an ultradistance trail venture and those fortunate few should consider themselves lucky.

For me, ultrarunning is a microcosm of life itself: It contains the drama, the struggle, the joy, and the redemption that makes life worth living. It brings the best in the human spirit.
—Stephanie Ehret, "Blow Up, Break Down," in *Marathon & Beyond*

To help survive the mentally tough times through which ultra trail runners inevitably pass, use a strong training foundation. Call upon the hundreds of miles you have logged and convince yourself that your body is physically capable of making it through the miles. Commit to the finish without dismissing injury- or death-related symptoms, distinguishing them from feelings of discomfort, temporary illness, and low motivation.

The beauty of the trail is also a good motivator if your goal is to finish an ultra. Rather than running for a certain time or place goal, Helen Klein, an age-group world-record holder in a number of ultradistances, recommends running trail ultras for the peacefulness they instill. Although runners need to be more self-sufficient and focused for trail ultras, Klein recognizes that "the trails are kinder to your body and your mind. Nature somehow helps you run relaxed and alert at the same time."

[B]ecause most ultras in the United States are on trails rather than roads, the ultrarunner will usually benefit from running on a forgiving dirt surface. In addition, thanks to the softer surfaces of trails, runners can often increase mileage without the expected increase in running injuries.
—Richard Benyo, editor of *Marathon & Beyond*

Peter Bakwin recognizes the importance of setting short-term goals in order to reach a larger objective. He recommends giving oneself certain rewards—like slowing down, walking, eating, drinking—every half hour or so. To him, it is too much of an emotional strain to try to say "only eighteen hours to go" and stay motivated. Breaking an ultra down into segments works much better if the runner can think, "only twenty minutes more and then I can walk for a minute."

Breaking an ultra into different subsections also makes it more manageable. Try staying focused on only the next aid station and then set a new goal when you reach the station. This "one step at a time" approach helps to get through bouts of pain, depression, sleepiness, hunger, nausea, and cramps while out on long trail runs and races.

Talking with other runners may also help when struggling in a trail ultra. By tackling the long miles together, fellow ultrarunners can motivate one another to finish. As Ian Torrence says, "Remember everyone else is hurting too. It helps to talk to other runners and commiserate with them." Family and friends along the course can also serve as a reward and moral support.

Visualization is another tool that helps ultrarunners to make it through tough times on the trail. Fix in your mind an image of yourself at the finish and think about how good you will feel when you cross the line. Conversely, if that carrot does not work to motivate you, think about how you will feel later if you drop out of the ultra and use the stick trick.

However much visualization may help, you still have to run the race. Dana Miller, five-time winner of the Wasatch 100 in Utah, liked a quote from multiday ultrarunner Yiannos Kouros so much that he wore it on his shirt when he won the race in 1990 (setting a course record at the time). Kouros's inspirational statement was: "You cannot be at the finish line only in your mind because the others will not be able to see it." To Miller, the phrase means that you can only be where you are physically in a race—not daydreaming about some finish line. Miller has realized that his slips, twisted ankles, and sticks in the eye usually happened when he lost focus and started thinking too far ahead.

A Psychological Analysis of
Trail Runners

*By Beth Darnall, PhD in Psychiatry at the Oregon Health and Science
University and a competitive runner for over twenty years*

Every sport has its own unique culture, replete with customs surrounding fashion, lingo, and various types of behavior. All of this is apparent not only within the sport scene itself, but bleeds over into the everyday lives of those athletes who identify with that sport. Notice how gymnasts wear their hair and makeup a certain way as a distinct hallmark of the gymnast culture. One can often spot a dancer in a group and identify her as such, based on subcultural markers. Group customs are an interesting phenomenon that lead to the chicken-and-egg question: Is one attracted to a sport because the sport's subculture is a good match with one's personality, or does one engage in a sport and then slowly conform to the sport's culture based on frequency of exposure?

Perhaps the greatest and most immediate distinction I found between road running and trail running was that the latter introduced a large helping of unpredictability into what is otherwise a relatively predictable sport. The most obvious manifestation of this idea is the terrain, the characteristic of the ground surface engendered in the moniker of both forms of running. There are few surprises in road running; you generally have a smooth and relatively clean synthetic surface of cement or pavement. In trail running, varying degrees of technicality and difficulty are associated with different trails, but the common denominator is that the trail runner deals with the earth, not a waterproof impervious hardtop. Add a bit of precipitation and you've got mud, slush, and clay, none of which are conducive to PRs or fast splits. The same could be said of the frequent inclines and winding courses of many trails that make for some slow going.

When trail running, you not only intimately traverse the bare skin of the earth, you also pierce the nature of a lush forest, of grassy hills, or of sandy desert. You hear people weary of the world say they need to "get away from it all," meaning perhaps that they need to indulge in an expensive vacation. Astute trail runners know they can literally get away from it all via any given trail. In this sense and in this state, trail running can be seen as the celebratory dance of life and spirit; both our own and that which surrounds us.

Where you choose to run—your choice of terrain, your choice of venue—says something about who you are. Do you prefer to run on a flat, paved course and compare your splits each week, or do you run on a different rocky trail each day, preferably at a time when the light makes the views that much more beautiful? The former runner may have serious 10K ambitions and may find comfort in the training struc- ture that quickly yields information reflecting monitored progress. The latter runner may have serious competitive ambitions as well, but fur- ther delights in the nature and the variety of the trails.

CHAPTER 4

Trail Training at Every Distance

Once you have reached a comfort level with trails and have developed proper trail running technique, your next focus is likely to be on accelerating your pace and becoming a stronger, more agile, and efficient trail runner. Whether your goal is to simply learn to run a steady pace on varying terrain or improve your time in a trail race, the training techniques contained in this chapter will prove invaluable.

Whereas road training is a more straightforward, linear endeavor, trail training is multidimensional because it blends lateral motion with forward movement. To adapt your training routine to accommodate the varying terrain of trails, you will need to focus on strengthening your

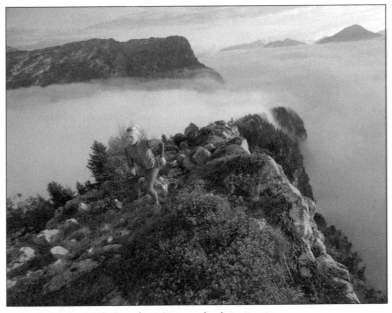

Trails can lead to that feeling of running on a cloud. Stephan/Gripmaster

stabilizing muscles and improving balance. Similarly, because you are bound to encounter hills as a trail runner, you should consider the benefits of including training workouts that focus on strength, such as by running hill repeats. If you want to become a faster trail runner, consider improving your fitness by running intervals. Finally, you may want to hit the weight room and stretch. Strength training and stretching for trail running are addressed in Chapters 5 and 6, respectively.

Trail running is only one part of your life, and the question of how large a part it will play is one that you are likely to revisit. To be a "whole" trail runner, you will probably want to supplement your trail running with other recreational activities and balance your physical life with your family, career, and social life. You will also need to integrate recovery into your training regimen by blending active rest, cross training, or simply sitting on the couch. Depending on your particular trail running goals, consider integrating any or all of the following training techniques into your routine.

Although many of the training techniques discussed in this chapter apply to road running, with the exception of some trail-specific speed training, it is important to try to perform them on trails if your goal is to become a better, more accomplished trail runner. Yes, you may become a faster road runner by doing speed work on the track; but that speed does not always transfer to trails, where you will be forced to use a different stride, constantly adjust your tempo, and maintain control while altering your course to stay upright.

DISTANCE TRAINING

If you seek to run or race a course of a certain length, then training for that distance will be a mandatory building block in your trail training regimen. Incorporating long runs into weekly training will help your body adjust physiologically to the increased body stress by generating more bone calcium deposits and building more and stronger leg muscles and connective tissue. Building up weekly mileage improves your aerobic capacity and helps to build up a base, upon which you can mix speed and strength training runs into your schedule.

Heart Rate Training Techniques

Different types of training techniques can achieve different targets of fitness and performance. To optimize Vo_2 max, it is necessary to stress the body's oxygen delivery and processing systems while performing the specific type of activity that you seek to improve.

To improve lactate threshold, an athlete needs to exercise at approximately 70 to 90 percent of maximum heart rate, depending on fitness level. Subjectively, threshold pace is a pace that is tolerable but slightly uncomfortable. Unless otherwise indicated, it is important to maintain threshold pace during the course of a workout.

Certain types of heart rate monitors are designed to measure a person's maximum heart rate during a workout while maintaining a historical record of that rate so it can be compared to prior VO_2 max training sessions. Advanced heart rate monitors allow a person to monitor workload by programming a target rate zone. Other heart rate monitors alert the user with an audible alarm if their heart rate drops below or rises above the established rate zone.

Longer training runs enable your body to cope with high mileage by breaking down fats for fuel and becoming more biomechanically efficient. Psychologically, long runs teach you to cope with and understand fatigue. During lengthy training runs one frequently experiences what can become an emotional roller coaster. It is useful to become familiar with how you respond under such circumstances, especially if you are training for a longer distance trail race. Long runs also help build confidence as a measure of progress. And, perhaps best, these runs become adventures into uncharted territory, allowing you to explore new stretches of trails and see new sights.

Train for Time

When Chad Ricklefs was asked about his weekly training mileage for an upcoming Leadville Trail 100 (which he went on to win), he responded, "between seventeen and twenty a week." Ricklefs was not talking about miles; he was talking about *hours!*

While Ricklefs's example may be somewhat intimidating, it illustrates how trail runners should measure their training effort by their total time spent running rather than distance. The measure of time is often more meaningful than distance because, assuming a relatively constant level of exertion, unlike the constant of time, the distance covered will vary dramatically depending on factors such as changes in grade, altitude, footing, and weather conditions. Whether the time you spend running is one hour a week or twenty hours a week, it is better to measure the workload by time rather than by trying to convert that effort to distance.

Some simple advice for those converting from roads to trails—especially for those who keep a log to record time, distance, and pace—is to forget about training distance or, if you know the distance of a trail, leave your watch behind when you go for a training run. Since trail running is invariably slower than road running, you will only get frustrated if you make the common mistake of comparing your trail pace with your road or track pace.

A central reason so many of us run trails is to escape tedious calculations, so go ahead and free yourself from either distance or time constraints and just run and enjoy, particularly during your initial exposure to trail running. Tap into the wonderful feeling of breezing by brush and trees as you flow up and down hills and maneuver sharp corners with skill and agility. You can always fret about your pace as you develop your trail skills and speed.

Building Time (and Distance)

When building up to a particular goal of either distance or time, it is wise to dedicate one day of the week to a considerably longer training run. If you base your trail running training on the premise that long runs are primarily a function of time rather than ground covered, you should keep training runs close to the amount of time you think it will take to run your target distance. For example, if you are training to complete a 5-mile trail run in the near future, you might set your training run for forty-five minutes. If, however, you are training for a trail marathon or ultramarathon, you probably want to keep your distance training to somewhat less than the time it will take you to complete the race distance. Those who train for a 100K or 100-miler usually do not exceed seven- or eight-hour runs on their "long" training days, even though they will be running for thirty or more hours on the ultra race day(s). Doing back-to-back long runs helps ultramarathoners simulate the stress that they'll be putting their bodies through on race day. Some also use cross training, such as cycling, and log a handful of hours on foot only to transition directly to the bike for several more hours for a prolonged training session with less mechanical impact but continued effort for the body, thus reducing the likelihood of injury.

Kami Semick

Kami Semick, one of the nation's top ultrarunners, who is based in Bend, Oregon, shares some of her training insights for ultra training:

Much has been written on training for the marathon distance. Less has been written about training for ultra distances. I'm going to guess there are two reasons for the lack of cohesive agreement on how to train for ultras:

1. Races vary by such a huge amount that there really is no standard that could apply to "ultras" as a whole. Hardrock and World Cup 100K are completely different.

2. Individuals vary greatly in how much their bodies can handle from a quality and quantity perspective.

Here are my guidelines that I abide by when putting together a training program for a key race:

1. Match your training terrain on long runs to the terrain of your goal race.

2. Include at least one day of rest per week.

- Our bodies become stronger not when we are running, but when we rest. Allow your body to adapt to the training by taking one day a week of rest. If you're really antsy, go swim.

- On recovery run days, really recover. Don't be tempted to run a faster pace because your friend is turning a recovery run into a tempo workout. Do what's right for you.

- Your recovery pace should feel easy. You should be able to hold a lengthy conversation. I try to keep my recovery runs less than seventy-five minutes.

3. Include at a minimum one quality workout per week.

- For my bread and butter quality workout, I do a tempo run. Tempo runs are done at a "comfortably hard" pace, a pace that you know you can sustain for whatever period of time you have allocated. A tempo run is not a time trial and should not wipe you out. At the beginning of the season, I will start my tempo run at about twenty minutes. I like to do tempo runs on a flat, measurable course so that I can track my pace per mile. Then, over the course of the season, I add five minutes onto my tempo run every two to three weeks. I build up to a max of sixty minutes. Sometimes I play with the time, and do two twenty-minute sessions with five minutes recovery in between instead of a forty-minute tempo. You could also do three fifteen-minute sessions with three minutes recovery in between. Play with the tempo time and your recovery time to change up your workout.

4. Work on core strength.

- This doesn't mean doing a bunch of crunches. Your core is everything in between your quads and your shoulders. I've found Pilates to be a great core strengthener. I'm not motivated enough to put together my own core routine, so I attend at least one class a week, although my goal is always two.

TEN-WEEK DISTANCE TRAINING SCHEDULE

The following schedule should serve as a sample for building a foundation from which a beginning trail runner might train to complete a 10K trail race. The schedule is based on a goal of finishing the 10K in an hour. If you are building up to do a shorter distance—a 5K—then adjust the numbers by reducing the time by approximately 30 percent. If you are a more experienced runner or can maintain a faster pace, then adjust by reducing it proportionally and run for the allotted time at a faster pace. Alternatively, if you are training for a half, full, or ultramarathon, then make the runs longer. For those approaching trail running from a developed cardiovascular fitness base, you can generally add more workouts each week and increase the exercise times based on the workload with which you are comfortable. Your weekend runs can be longer than those listed.

Week One: Monday, Wednesday, and Friday run, jog, or walk twenty to thirty minutes; Saturday or Sunday run, jog, or walk thirty to forty minutes, with the other day a rest day. Tuesday and Thursday should be days of active rest or cross training.

Week Two: Monday, Wednesday, and Friday run, jog, or walk twenty-five to thirty-five minutes with less walking than week one; Saturday or Sunday run, jog, or walk thirty-five to forty-five minutes, with the other day a rest day. Tuesday and Thursday should be days of active rest or cross training.

Week Three: Monday, Wednesday, and Friday run, jog, or walk twenty-five to forty minutes with less walking than week two; Saturday or Sunday run, jog, or walk forty to fifty minutes, with the other day a rest day. Tuesday and Thursday should be days of active rest or cross training. If, however, you feel strong at the end of your run on Monday or Wednesday, either (but not both) Tuesday or Thursday could be used for a short run—not to exceed twenty minutes—in lieu of cross training.

Week Four: Monday, Wednesday, and Friday run or jog thirty to forty minutes (by this point in the training schedule you should only use walking for ascents); Saturday or Sunday run or jog forty-five to fifty minutes, with the other day a rest day. Tuesday and Thursday should be days of active rest or cross training. If you feel strong at the end of your run on Monday or Wednesday, either (but not both) Tuesday or Thursday could be used for a short run—not to exceed twenty-five minutes—in lieu of or in addition to the cross training.

Week Five: Monday, Wednesday, and Friday run or jog thirty-five to forty-five minutes; Saturday or Sunday run or jog fifty to fifty-five minutes, with the other day a rest day. Tuesday and Thursday should be days of active rest or cross training. If you feel strong at the end of your run on Monday or Wednesday, either Tuesday or Thursday could be used for a short run—not to exceed thirty minutes—in lieu of or in addition to the cross training.

Week Six: Monday, Wednesday, and Friday run or jog thirty-five to fifty minutes; Saturday or Sunday run or jog fifty to sixty minutes, with the other day a rest day. Tuesday and Thursday should be days of active rest or cross training. If, however, you feel strong at the end of your run on Monday or Wednesday, Tuesday and/or Thursday could be used for a short run—not to exceed thirty minutes—in lieu of or in addition to the cross training.

Week Seven: Monday, Wednesday, and Friday run or jog forty to fifty minutes; Saturday or Sunday run or jog fifty-five to sixty-five minutes, with the other day a rest day. The rest can be active rest. Tuesday and Thursday should be days of active rest or cross training. If, however, you feel strong at the end of your run on Monday or Wednesday, Tuesday and/or Thursday could be used for a short run—not to exceed thirty-five minutes—in lieu of or in addition to the cross training.

Week Eight: Monday, Wednesday, and Friday run or jog forty-five to fifty minutes; Saturday or Sunday run or jog fifty-five to sixty-five minutes, with the other day a rest day. The rest can be active rest. Tuesday and Thursday should be days of active rest or cross training. If, however, you feel strong at the end of your run on Monday or Wednesday, Tuesday and/or Thursday could be used for a short run—not to exceed thirty-five minutes—in addition to the cross training.

Week Nine: Monday, Wednesday, and Friday run or jog forty-five to fifty-five minutes; Saturday or Sunday run or jog sixty to seventy-five minutes, with the other day a rest day. The rest should be active rest. Tuesday and Thursday should be days of active rest or cross training. If, however, you feel strong at the end of your run on Monday or Wednesday, Tuesday and/or Thursday could be used for a short run—not to exceed thirty-five minutes—in lieu of or in addition to the cross training.

Week Ten: Monday, Wednesday, and Friday run or jog forty-five to fifty-five minutes; Saturday or Sunday run or jog sixty-five to seventy-five minutes, with the other day a rest day. Tuesday and Thursday should be days of active rest or cross training. If, however, you feel strong at the end of your run on Monday or Wednesday, Tuesday and/or Thursday could be used for a short run—not to exceed thirty-five minutes—in lieu of or in addition to the cross training.

Depending on the ultimate distance goal, you will eventually want to work up to close to the goal distance (or at least half the distance, if you are training for a race longer than a 50-miler). To get to that point, you may want to set aside between one day every two weeks to two days a week for long runs, depending on your goal, experience, fitness background, and resistance to injury.

Some runners prefer to run two back-to-back relatively long days, especially on weekends when their schedules are more accommodating. This latter training method, known as a "brick workout," is common among ultramarathoners, who must condition their bodies to perform while tired and stressed. Newer runners should not try brick workouts until they are both comfortable with trails and are confident that their bodies will be able to withstand two days of long runs without breaking down or suffering injuries.

Beware of the Forgiving Trail

Because the forgiving surface of trails may allow one to run relatively injury free, newer trail runners are often lulled into prematurely building up their distance base with long runs. Whether performed on road or trail, distance often leads to injury, burnout, or susceptibility to illness. Depending on age, experience with endurance athletics in general, and one's running history, it is better to increase your mileage or time running by no more than 5 to 10 percent per week.

Even if you increase your mileage base gradually, do not forfeit quality for quantity. Many runners succumb to the unhealthy game of comparing weekly mileage with either their previous weeks' or that of other runners. Junk miles are just that. Depending on your objectives, it is usually better to run fewer miles with fresher legs and at a more intense pace, than to slog through miles merely to rack them up in your logbook.

One way to check the quality of your miles is to wear a heart rate monitor, and couple the distance of your runs with the goal of staying within your training zone at a steady pace. If you find your heart rate consistently rising above or falling below that target rate as you tack on the miles, then that is a sign you are overtraining, and it is unlikely you will derive much benefit from those miles unless you are training for ultradistance.

SPEED TRAINING

Building up one's distance base should naturally help to increase running speed—but only to a certain extent. To really pick up your pace and break through your personal speed barrier, you should run fast. Running at a faster pace helps to improve both cardiovascular fitness and biomechanical efficiency. This section, however, is aimed at those who find it more exhilarating to push their limits, who enjoy the feeling of rushing along a wooded path, and who appreciate the fitness improvements that result from challenging themselves.

Beyond velocity, speed training—whether through intervals, repeats, tempo runs, fartleks (see below), or other means—has positive physiological effects. Pushing the pace at regular intervals with rests in between forces muscles and energy systems to adapt to the more strenuous effort needed to run faster. The body does this by improving the flow of blood to muscles, increasing the number of capillaries in muscle fiber, stimulating your muscles to increase their myoglobin and mitochondria content, and raising aerobic enzyme activity to allow muscles to produce more energy aerobically.

Speed training also provides a mental edge. If you are already familiar with the stress and burning sensation known to many as "pain and suffering" that accompany pushing at a faster-than-normal pace during training, you will be able to draw from that experience psychologically and dig deeper into your reserves when needed during a race. Speed training on trails also forces you to push your comfort level with respect to the risk of falling or otherwise losing control on difficult terrain. Pushing the envelope helps establish a sense of confidence that is crucial to running difficult sections, especially descents, at speed.

Since speed training is an advanced form of training, it should not be introduced into your routine until you establish a consistent training base. Beginning trail runners should start by becoming comfortable with running on trails before they endeavor to run those trails quickly. It may be wise to do faster workouts on more tame trails with dependable footing, such as dirt roads, or even a track or road. Only if you are a very advanced trail runner should you attempt to do speed training on technical trails, where the potential for injury caused by a sprained or rolled ankle, tripping over an obstacle, or other casualty is much greater.

Do We Love Pain?

Not long ago, I posted the question on a blog site: "Are we endurance athletes driven by the solipsistic need for self-validation, as in, 'we hurt, therefore we are'; or is it that we love the pain and exertion and, therefore, more is better?"

The answers were quite edifying so I thought I'd share them:

—Personally, I love it—the pain, I mean. But most importantly, I view the pain as the engine to drive me to reach my goals. In other words, I know I'm hurting because I'm on hour four of a six-hour effort and that I'm that much closer to seeing nature in full effect. Or, that the pain is getting me through a technical uphill section. The pain is an indication that I'm do-ing!

—I train so I don't hurt any more.

—I tend to agree; when I was most prepared to race, pain wasn't that much of a factor. The validation came in competing against others.

—I was getting a massage last night, and the therapist asked, "You *do* work your body hard, don't you? What is your motivation?" I didn't know what to say, mainly because my face was being shoved into the hole as he stretched my calf and it was hard to talk anyway . . . but he made me think. I don't know that I have a good answer, but I agree that training is to avoid future pain. I also know that I absolutely *love* being out in the wilderness, and the harder I train, the more time I am able to spend in that environment.

—It's all about the balance. You feel *so* good afterwards because you suffered through the pain during it. The sweetness of completing something wouldn't be the same if it was easy to do. Being in pain, working through it, and finishing bring the accomplishment more meaning.

—I say it's like most things in life: combo platter.

—I don't love pain . . . but it makes me stronger, and in that way it helps me achieve my goals. I think the key to the answer lies within our personal goals.

—Balance. For me it's all about the three-part teeter totter: sport, family, work. Each causes (good) pain the harder you try at it, and all must be in balance to make each truly meaningful.

—Maybe we like the pain. Maybe we're wired that way. Because without it, I don't know, maybe we just wouldn't feel real. What's that saying? "Why do I keep hitting myself with a hammer? Because it feels so good when I stop." I can't take credit for the quote, but it seems somewhat appropriate.

—I love it and think that more is fun but moderation is the key to longevity and health. I'm enjoying my Boston Marathon hangover. Pain is relative. I just wish I could recover quicker!

—If pain feels good, if pain = pleasure, then is it really pain? But I am proud to be one of the finish-line crossers so maybe pain = proud.

—It's not the pain that's enjoyable, it's the feeling of accomplishment and daily reinforcement that your body is adapting—getting stronger and/or faster. Pain is a reminder that you pushed hard. We need to be more aware about the weakest point in our body, as that seems to break first. Strengthen the weakest part to keep the rest in balance.

—So many times I've been asked if I love pain. Or, why do I put myself through all this "insane training and criminal early (very early) morning runs?" And I have questioned myself, too: why? I love pain, I do, it makes me feel *alive*! It makes me feel I trained, I paid my dues, I have a right to be where I am. Too crazy? Maybe.

Speed Workouts

The following sections discuss some recommended forms of speed training. Each exercise targets a different kind of result. Depending on your particular trail running goals and strengths, you may want to focus on some forms of speed training over others. You should feel free to mix and match the various speed training methods based on the returns and benefits you get from each and on how they fit into your training schedule and performance goals.

If you choose to work speed training into your weekly training schedule, be sure to do so on a gradual basis, starting with one day of speed a week and keeping the intensity to a moderate level. It is common to reserve a day in the middle of the week for speed work because that timing spaces out the effort and allows for recovery from and preparation for long weekend runs. Because speed training is both physically and emotionally draining, it is important to go into a session feeling strong and to allow ample rest after a tough speed workout. Many runners find that doing speed workouts with a group helps them stay motivated and disciplined. Competition serves to increase the intensity of the training, but the workout should not become a full-on race, unless that is the goal for the session.

Intervals

Although interval training improves leg speed, its primary goal is cardio-vascular—to optimize lactate threshold. As an anaerobic training tool, intervals are designed to increase one's ability to maintain a fast pace for a longer period of time. Without an improvement in lactate threshold, you will be unable to run or race a substantial distance at a faster pace than the rate at which your body can comfortably use oxygen, thereby causing lactate to form in the bloodstream. Intervals help to raise the level at which the body begins the lactate production process, so that you can run faster and longer without feeling muscles burn or cramp. Upon developing a substantial training base of endurance, strength intervals allow acceleration of pace and an increase in overall running fitness.

Intervals are usually measured in terms of time rather than distance, especially if run on hilly or rugged trails. During the "on" or hard-effort segments of interval training, you should work hard enough to go anaerobic (i.e., faster than your lactate threshold, which is approximately 70 to 90 percent of your maximum heart rate, so that the body goes into oxygen debt). Although not an all-out sprint, the pace should be uncomfortable. During the "off" or recovery segments you are allowed to repay some of the oxygen debt, but not all of it. The rest period should be sufficiently short so that you are "on" again before full recovery.

An interval workout may be a series of equal on-and-off intervals and recovery periods, or a mix of different length intervals and recoveries. For example, you might run six intervals of four minutes each interspersed with three-minute recoveries. Alternatively, you might mix it up with five-, four-, three-, two-, three-, four-, and five-minute intervals each separated by a three-minute recovery.

Intervals can be as long as six minutes and as short as thirty seconds. Run longer intervals if training for longer distances, and run shorter intervals if speed is your goal. The off, or recovery, period between intervals is an active rest that ranges between jogging and moderate running. Recovery time should be a little shorter than the time of the interval preceding it. To improve the value of your interval sessions, strive to decrease the length of the recovery period relative to the time of the hard effort. In addition to recoveries between the intervals, any interval workout should integrate a substantial warm-up before and cooldown after running at or above lactate threshold pace.

Hill Repeats and Repetition Workouts

Hill repeats resemble intervals, except that leg speed and strength are emphasized more than lactate threshold, although "repeats" also offer a good lactate threshold workout because you push hard to go anaerobic on the climb. Generally speaking, repeat workouts are designed for biomechanical and physiological improvement more than for cardiovascular benefits. Hill repeats are intended to hone your climbing skills and make you a stronger runner by taxing the muscular system.

Like intervals, repeats are run at or faster than lactate threshold pace; however, each interval is shorter in length than in a standard interval workout. Typically, repeats last two minutes or less. Since the focus is muscle strength improvement rather than cardio fitness, the active rest between repeats should be long enough to recharge the muscles and prepare for the next repeat at or above lactate threshold. In short, if you run a two-minute repeat and need three minutes to recover, take the full three minutes. You want to recover enough to make each repeat interval sufficiently intense to realize the full benefits of the exercise. Run each interval at a pace that you can maintain through the entire repeat workout. Do not push so hard during early repeats that you are unable to finish the rest of the workout.

Tempo Runs

Imagine a spectrum, with repeats, which focus on biomechanics and muscular strength buildup at one end; intervals, which focus on a combination of

Effect of Hills on Heart Rate

The relationship between heart rate and vertical ascent rate is direct and linear. You should expect to see a tandem rise in the two rates ascending hills or mountains. Imagine starting at the bottom of a long hill that takes you thirty minutes to ascend at a relaxed pace. Now, assume you run the same hill in only twenty minutes at a more rigorous pace. Your ascent rate at the rigorous pace will be one-third faster than the ascent rate at the relaxed pace, and there should be a corresponding relationship between your heart rates (although your average heart rate at the rigorous pace may not be exactly one-third higher than at the relaxed pace).

Depending on how hill training is performed, it can translate to more speed through better economy, greater strength, optimized VO_2 max, and improved lactate threshold. Hill repeats help to optimize VO_2 max, whereas longer steadier hill training improves lactate threshold.

Another type of heart rate training is performed in hilly settings that offer steady climbs and descents. The objective of this particular training is to maintain your heart rate in a certain zone for the entire workout (excluding the warm-up and cooldown phases), regardless of whether you are on an ascent, descent, or flat. Certain heart rate monitors are particularly suited for tracking these kinds of hill workouts because they will alert you if you fall above or below your predetermined zone. To attain a steady heart rate workout, you should maintain a consistent, even pace on the flats, back off the pace as the grades become steeper, and push yourself during descents.

lactate threshold and biomechanics in the middle; and tempo runs at the other end, which emphasize lactate threshold or cardiovascular fitness.

Repeats	Intervals	Tempo Runs
Biomechanics/Strength		Cardio/Lactate Threshold

Tempo runs are sustained efforts at an even pace, usually lasting about twenty to forty minutes, although those training for longer distances may do tempo runs that stretch to ninety minutes. The pace should be a lactate threshold pace—which, again, is approximately 70 to 90 percent of your maximum heart rate. The pace is one that could be maintained for about an hour, if racing. Since the goal of tempo training is to maintain a steady pace with consistent leg turnover, run tempos on a trail or dirt road that is relatively flat with good footing.

Tempo runs should include a warm-up and cooldown at a comfortable pace. If the tempo workout involves training partners, be careful to not turn the session into a race or time trial. To prevent that from occurring, wear a heart rate monitor and set it to sound an alarm if the heart rate rises above lactate threshold rate. Because tempo runs are physiological workouts, the goal is to run at a certain effort rather than to cover a certain distance. Depending on terrain, weather, or how rested you feel beginning a tempo run, the pace may vary, but the body should nevertheless be working at threshold level throughout the workout.

Because considerable concentration and focus is required to maintain a steady lactate threshold pace for twenty minutes or longer, runners frequently find themselves a bit tired, both physically and mentally, the next day or two after a tempo workout. If that is the case, take a day of active rest or work a recovery run into your schedule. It may even be advisable to take the next day off to rest up and maintain trail running vigor.

Remember when you were a kid, playing in your schoolyard on one of those long, magical summer evenings that lingered on and on? . . . You would sprint, then rest, then sprint again, looking over your shoulder and laughing a rib-busting, out-of-breath laugh as you tried to stay a step ahead of your friends. . . . That kind of joyful play in running that we all experienced as children can be recaptured in a fartlek session.
—Michael Sandrock, *Running Tough*

Fartleks
Fartlek is Swedish for "speed play." Scandinavians, known for their trail running prowess and long history in the sport, pioneered the art of

running fast on trails. Fartleks are creative workouts that weave a variety of paces into the same run: It is unstructured fast running over varying terrain with interspersed periods of recovery. Although fartleks can be performed solo, they are often run as a group in single file with the leader setting the pace—sometimes sprinting, sometimes jogging, sometimes walking, at other times simply running. Because the pace of a fartlek often varies with the terrain, these invigorating workouts are most successful if run on trails that offer a mix of short and long hills and plenty of turns and obstacles. As testament to the loose, definition-defying nature of this kind of somewhat random workout, there are T-shirts that say FARTLEK: IT'S A RUNNER'S THING.

Fartleks offer a fun alternative to more standardized, timed speed workouts. Because they lack any regimented order, fartleks can reinject zip into a training routine that has grown boring, or introduce some excitement when running feels lethargic. The pacesetter can rotate, and faster runners may loop back to pick up stragglers to keep the fartlek group intact. A fartlek run can be as short as fifteen minutes or as long as a couple of hours, although they typically last between a half hour and an hour.

To capture some benefits of a fartlek when running alone, throw in some surges to get some speed training. Surges are short blasts of speed worked into a training run to accentuate a transition in the trail, such as near the top of a hill or when reaching the bottom of a hill and beginning a climb.

Striders and Accelerations

Another way to mix training with a little speed is to integrate striders or accelerations into your routine. An excellent time to do this is at the end of a trail run, just before the cooldown. A strider is usually run at a fast running pace, just under or even finishing with a sprint. Place the emphasis on high knee lifts and getting a full kick off each step so as to cover as much ground as possible without overstriding. When striding, think of sprinters warming up on a track, swinging their arms and lifting their knees in an accentuated manner. Accelerations resemble striders but begin more slowly and end in a full sprint.

Striders and accelerations are usually performed on flat, soft surfaces such as grassy parks, playing fields, or dirt roads. If striders or accelerations are run on grass or sand, try removing your shoes so as to work on the muscle tone of the lower legs and feet. By taking away the structure of shoes, the smaller supporting muscles in your lower legs and feet have a chance to develop while you are invigorated by the freedom and lightness of bare feet. Strider and acceleration distances should range between 50 and 100 meters, allowing for an additional 10 meters to get started and 20 to 30 to slow down.

"Off-Trail" Speed Training

It is not always necessary to do all speed training on trails. In fact, it can occasionally be more effective to perform some speed training sessions on a track, dirt, or even paved roads. Depending on where you live and the types of trails to which you have access, it may be a lot easier to do speed training off the trails, reserving the trip to trails for longer runs.

Road and track are better suited for certain types of speed training. Tempo runs, where the focus is on a steady pace, and repeats, where the emphasis is on leg turnover, should be performed on flatter, more dependable surfaces. Roads or tracks are certainly easier than the trail for these types of workouts, especially when the trails are icy or muddy.

Track sessions tend to be highly efficient. Perhaps it is the lane lines or bends of the turns, but there is something about running on a track that creates a feeling of running fast. That feeling may well convert to actual speed, which means a more effective speed session. Tracks are also convenient because they are measured for pacing. If one wants to do repeats or intervals and maintain a set pace, going to the track is an efficient alternative to the trail.

In addition to selecting the appropriate speed workout and venue to perform the session, also take the weather into consideration. If it is snowy, icy, muddy, or particularly windy, it may not be possible to get a good speed workout outside. Depending on training needs and personal preferences, train inside and run a set of repeats or intervals on the treadmill, or work on leg turnover by spinning on an indoor bike trainer. Skipping rope is another alternative that can simulate a speed workout. Many trail runners are adamantly opposed to such mechanical alternatives and insist on running outside, regardless of the weather. That is fine and well, but they then must be willing to either forego speed training sessions when the weather is particularly nasty or attempt to do them under unfavorable conditions.

RECOVERY, REST, AND COMMON SENSE

More is not always better. This is sometimes the most difficult lesson for enthusiastic trail runners to fully absorb. However, failure to learn this lesson may well lead to overuse injury or chronic suboptimal performance. The best ultrarunners know that some rest, even if only active rest through cross training, enhances running performance. Just as the need exists to integrate recovery and rest into repeat or interval training to get the most from each repeat or interval, periods of recovery and rest should be integrated into an overall training schedule. It often takes more discipline to take a day off than to go hard or long.

With proper recovery and rest, trail runners are able to attack hard days and make them worthwhile. Without recovery and rest, the pace of hard runs and easy runs will be approximately the same, and very little benefit will result from either. You may boast of having put in a solid month of 120-mile weeks yet show little to no benefit from such high mileage. Alternatively, a runner who puts in as few as 30 to 40 miles a week in three or four runs can show tremendous progress if each of those runs serves a particular training purpose. Design the easy days to accomplish a purpose, and transfer any pent-up energy to the hard or long days to really make those workouts count toward improvement.

Recovery and rest periods should come between repeats and intervals, between hard workouts, and before and after races. The use of recovery and rest also applies on a macro level, such as scheduling a particular season or year so as to build up to a specific running goal. You might want to pick a race as far off as a year, then train with that race in mind, perhaps running several "training" races geared to preparing for the target race.

If you are the type who is likely to overdo it, keep a running log or journal that tracks your daily runs, noting time, effort, mileage, and other pertinent factors such as weather, cross-training activities, sleep, diet, workload, emotional state, stress level, terrain, and, if you know them, altitude and heart rate. Those daily entries will force you to face the question of whether you are doing quality runs as opposed to sheer quantity (junk miles, as they are often called). The diary will also give an indication of whether you are overtraining. And when you notice progress in your running, you will be in a better position to recall and evaluate what factors worked to produce that success.

Another alternative for those who lack the discipline for proper recovery and rest is to get a coach. Although not many coaches specialize in trail training, a good running coach will be able to help you develop a customized training schedule that takes into consideration your personal strengths and weaknesses. A coach should also help integrate recovery days and rest into your training.

To ensure that easy days or recovery runs are not overly strenuous, arrange to run with someone who is willing to run with you at a moderate pace. Avoid running with someone who has a proclivity to pick it up or with whom you tend to be competitive. Consider running without a watch, or wear a heart rate monitor that can be set to beep if you have exceeded a predetermined rate. Be open to the idea of walking ascents, stopping to stretch, or simply smelling the flowers and enjoying a vista.

Gathering Ye Roses

By Lisa Jhung, trail runner, snowshoer, and adventure racer based out of Boulder, Colorado

I was running on a popular hiking trail in Bryce Canyon National Park in Utah, when an older man who was walking with his wife yelled, "Slow down and smell the roses!"

I smiled and said, "I see them," and kept running.

While I appreciated the fellow's notion to share his viewpoint and his vantage point of the canyon, I smiled to myself at the revelation that followed.

I run everywhere I go. In Florence, Italy, I ran despite dumbfounded stares of locals and found a park in the hills with beautiful ancient statues that I never would have seen. I had one of the best trail runs of my life in Bali, Indonesia, discovering rice paddy fields, steep, lush cliffs, and hidden rivers. I've seen more roses by running than I ever would have by walking.

Running isn't a way to rush through life and race by the roses. It's not a competition to see who can run around the entire garden first. For me, trail running while I travel is a way to feed my hunger for exploration while doing something I love.

The roses are out there for all of us—walkers and runners—to enjoy. "Gather ye rosebuds while ye may," said poet Robert Herrick. I choose to gather them while running.

Periodization

The training principle of "periodization" (also called "phase" training) is based on the idea that an athlete can reach a performance peak by building up through a set of steps, each of which may last for weeks or months, depending on the starting point and where the athlete wants to be at the peak of the periodization training. Periodization training starts with a buildup or foundation period upon which is built a base of endurance and strength. From there, the athlete works on speed and endurance, incorporating distance, tempo runs, intervals, repeats, and fartleks. Once fitness and strength levels are sufficient to run the target distance at close to goal pace, the runner reorients the focus to speed work and turnover to tweak muscles for a fast pace. It is at this point that the athlete enters a recovery phase, also known as the "taper" period.

Within the big picture of a periodization schedule, one should be prepared to make microadjustments for recovery and rest in order to stave off overtraining or injury. Know your body and be aware of heightened heart rate; sleep problems; loss of appetite; tight or sore muscles, bones, or connective tissue; a short temper; a general lack of enthusiasm; or other symptoms of burnout. Get adequate sleep by developing a consistent sleep routine. Quality of rest is probably more important than quantity, and playing catch-up does not always work to restore your body to a rested state. Also be sure to eat a balanced diet with adequate calories and fluids to power you through each workout and the entire day.

Cross Training

Skills and strengths gained from cross training easily translate to trail running. All of the following can help make you a better trail runner: the limbering and strengthening of muscles that come from rock climbing; the lung capacity gained from Nordic skiing; the high-altitude endurance from mountaineering; the descending skills of mountain biking; the leg strength gained from snowshoeing; and the muscular balance gained from swimming.

Cross training also gives some perspective to trail running. Cross training can be used as "active rest," when one can feel good about not running while pursuing another discipline or developing new skills that enhance the trail running dimension. By becoming passionate about other athletic endeavors, a trail runner is more likely to take adequate time away from running when a recovery period is necessary to recuperate from an overuse injury or in order to avoid overuse. Knowing that there are alternatives to running trails certainly helps during a time of injury, boredom, or burnout from running.

Cross training is easily integrated into the trail running routine by substituting a different discipline for a running session or two each week. These cross-training sessions should be of equivalent intensity as the running would have been, as measured by heart rate, effort, and time. For example, after a long trail run on Sunday, replace the normal Monday recovery run of forty-five minutes with a forty-five-minute swim, bike, or Nordic ski session of equivalent effort.

Only when one begins exchanging a substantial percentage of running workouts for cross training will the cross training begin to detract

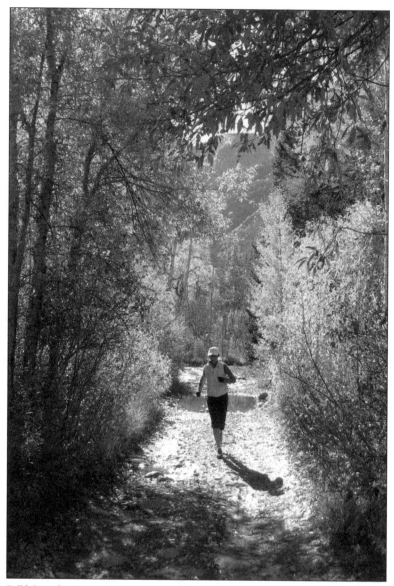

Fall foliage flanks a trail runner. Bernie Boettcher

from trail running performance. If the primary goal is to be a better trail runner, then it is probably important that a majority of the workouts be trail runs. The doctrine of "specificity of training" is an almost obvious principle: The best way to improve at an activity is to train by doing that activity. Trail runners should heed the specificity doctrine, but not to the point of ruling out beneficial cross-training workouts.

Depending on your trail running goals, cross training should complement and supplement running, but not supplant it. Although cross training is an excellent way of maintaining fitness while giving running muscles some time off, cross training should be thought of as active rest in that it should not be so strenuous or depleting that you are left too exhausted to pursue trail running training. Always exercise some caution when trying a new sport, because it is easy to strain muscles that are not trained for that specific activity. It is rather disappointing to spoil trail running training effort because of an injury resulting from a cross-training mishap.

Mind as Muscle

Engaging in yoga or meditation can play a useful part in the recovery and rest phase. Just because you are not running trails during time off does not mean that you must sacrifice the peace of mind gained from running in a beautiful place. Without lifting a foot, those who practice meditative arts are able to reach a state of equanimity and tranquility similar to that gained by running trails. Other restorative measures, if available, are saunas, hot tubs, or steam rooms. The benefits of sports massage are also likely to be worth the time and cost.

When determining the amount of recovery and rest that is needed, consider the impact of other life events and the effect that family, work, travel, social, and emotional lives have on training—and vice versa. The need may arise to run more or less during particularly stressful periods, regardless of the specific point in your training schedule. If emotionally drained, a long slow run in a scenic environment might replace what was supposed to be a hard hill repeat day.

Know yourself, set reasonable short- and long-term goals, and be willing to adjust them. Be flexible and avoid imposing on yourself a training partner's or someone else's goals. Every trail runner is an individual and responds to different types of training. What works for one trail runner might be a huge mistake for another. Be sensitive to all of your needs plus those of your family, friends, and coworkers.

A holistic approach to trail running will keep training in perspective. Yes, you need to respect the importance of adequate training, but do not forget the forest for the trees. You are better able to run the trail that leads through those trees if you are doing so from a more balanced place. In addition to proper form, fitness, strength, nutrition, and gear, you will become a better runner if you are happy with your family, work, and social life. Avoiding overtraining or chronic fatigue and approaching each run with fervor keeps you motivated and ensures quality training. You will also run more easily if not burdened by stress or lack of recovery, rest, and relaxation. Finally, common sense trumps total exhaustion, lasting pain, and serious injury.

Why Do We Run?

Jay Pozner ran track and cross-country at the University of Colorado and went on to finish second at the 1999 Leadville Trail 100 as a relative ultradistance rookie.

Why do we run? Is it for the wonderful reasons that so many of us appreciate, such as freedom of movement, getting in touch with our bodies, pushing performance, all the incredible things we see, or is it a self-esteem issue? It is scary that many runners have eating disorders, and having seen these kinds of problems, I attribute them to the paradox of self-analysis and questioning, even though introspection is one of the things I love about the sport.

Eating disorders are just the tip of the iceberg. I think that we can wrap ourselves into something so tight that it becomes a cocoon of safety. In my youth, I ran as an escape, but that was not always a productive thing. I used competition and workouts to hurt myself, cause pain, and in nearly any other self-destructive way I could. Because I was turning in some good race results, everyone supported it. Yet, if I was off a couple of races, my cocoon crumbled and my security was gone.

At the time I didn't run for the love of running. I ran for the need of acceptance. My point is that I know my experiences are often no different from others. Maybe it is a self-image issue, or the need to feel success, or any other thing that people run for, other than the true joy of running. What is most wonderful about my experience, though, is that as much as running was a way to hurt myself, it was also much of the cure. It is an expression, a love, an experience that I can share with myself and others.

I have taken my running to all levels throughout my life, and this issue is very real. I wonder sometimes if it takes someone who has been there to recognize it in others. That is why we really need to ask ourselves, "Why am I running?"

Training Your Mind

Trail running, with its diverse surface distractions, variable terrain, frequent hills, and susceptibility to the impact of weather, demands a certain amount of mental toughness and discipline of its participants. It is sometimes difficult to get out the door when the trails are muddy or icy or when there is a chill in the air. But if you are a devoted trail runner you can tap into the energy felt during a run, the release of tension that comes from running free and away from the paved world, and the massage it gives to your psyche. But motivation does not always come easily for everyone and sticking with a training schedule or getting through the tough days or miles is always a challenge.

If you find yourself lacking motivation, the following may help: Run in inclement weather and celebrate the cold, or wet, or depth of the snow, or mud. Change routes or run to the top of a mountain, along a creek or river, through a forest, or on a racecourse when there is no race. Run at a different time of day than normal or try running at night.

Turn your run into an adventure by throwing in some rock scrambling, a swim in a pond, or a river crossing. Make it a duathlon with some road or mountain biking to and from the trail.

You might also find it motivating to start your run with a certain goal, whether it be to run every step, make it higher up a mountain than ever before, keep your heart rate below or above a certain number of beats per minute, or run without thinking about anything other than the beauty around you. It may be fun to plan a running "date" or, alternatively, to throw in some silly running styles such as running backward, jumping from rock to rock, skipping, or hopping on one foot. Run with a group, go with a pet, or take a child in a running stroller and sing songs as you go. Finally, try taking some time to stop and smell the flowers, see some wildlife, or appreciate the views.

How the Pieces Fit

By Krissy Moehl

There are times when life creates opportunities that challenge us to ensure we are doing what we truly love. Whether it is the challenge that comes through a new or lost relationship, job, or move, we are faced with making decisions about what is important in life. My year of evaluating how and if running was to remain a key part of my life came in 2008.

I found myself in a new job in a new town, and running was not as present in my life as I had been used to. Since I started ultrarunning, I always had a lot of crossover with work and relationships somehow involving running. At times, nearly every aspect of my life was running. In my new setting, I bounced back and forth for a while between loving running one minute and wondering why the heck I own so many pairs of running shoes the next.

Some days I longed for more hours out on the trails, and others I found it difficult to even get out the door. I hardly signed up for races. I seemed to get sick or be out of town when invited on local long adventure runs; in fact, if it hadn't been for dawn patrol in Smith Rock, Ore., I don't know that I could have called myself a long distance runner.

The turning point came at the Grindstone 100. I went into that race tired from a lot of work travel, suffering from a head cold, and really questioning what the heck I was doing there. Thankfully, I had amazing support, a good day, and the time to reflect. I remembered how I just love being out on the trail. I often say there isn't a problem a long run can't fix, just sometimes the run has to be longer than others. I guess 100 miles was long enough this time.

During the Grindstone, I remembered that I do this because I want to, not because my job sends me to races (Oh, those were the days!) or because everyone around me is heading to the trails and/or races.

I love running through the woods, being outdoors, exploring new places with my own two feet, and being able to get to the less-traveled paths with less weight, impact, and time. Long distance running gives perspective, allows time to process, meditate, and reach understanding.

I love how raw running makes us. We are so vulnerable and exposed when running; sharing that time and experience with friends forms amazing bonds. Running creates a common ground between people who might otherwise not have anything in common.

I also love hearing "you got me into this." I have this theory that if you hang around me long enough I will get you to try an ultra. I still remember the first time someone told me that something I said had inspired him to try more. I love pacing and helping friends to the finish line. When people write or call to ask for my advice, I love being able to help or at least give a candid answer so they can decide whether or not it works for them. To me, the accomplishments of those I have turned on to the sport rank so much higher than my own, and the idea that what I do out there may make someone else break out of their normal routine and push their limits motivates me to try to do even more.

What an amazing experience and process to re-discover my passion, and to redefine something I have been doing for more than half of my life. It was not the first time running has taken new form for me and probably will not be the last. It was great to check in and make sure that this is still something I want to do, redefine why I do it, and realize what motivates me to continue.

CHAPTER 5

Strength Training for the Trail

Road runners are often pictured as being ectomorphs—somewhat bony humans with elongated muscles and perhaps a sunken chest. Without besmirching those who restrict their running to paved surfaces, it can be said that trail runners tend to be a bit more muscular and "shapely" than their roadie equivalents. Many reasons account for the differences, but an important one concerns the trail runner's proclivity to vary exercise and recreation routines with other sports, many of which build strength and use one's upper body.

When not running, you may want to gravitate toward other outdoor recreational activities, such as backpacking, rock climbing, swimming, road or mountain biking, kayaking, backcountry or Nordic skiing, or even horseback riding. These other disciplines build strength and draw on muscles that are used less or not often when running. Many trail runners alter their workouts to combine trail running and at least one other outdoor activity. For example, you might run to the base of a mountain to do some bouldering or bicycle to a trailhead and go for a run.

You can also complement and enhance running strength with resistance training. Given that trail running draws from a broad range of muscles, the balance derived from regularly hitting the weight room can have considerable performance-enhancing benefits, on and off the trail. Not only can one gain strength for speed and hill ascents through resistance training, but it serves to prevent injury, increase resting metabolism, align and balance muscles for improved biomechanics, and build tendon and ligament strength.

Given the numerous benefits from many types of resistance or weight-bearing exercise, this chapter outlines only a few approaches you might consider in a training routine. This is not *The Ultimate Guide to Weightlifting,* so to learn proper form and method, seek the advice of a

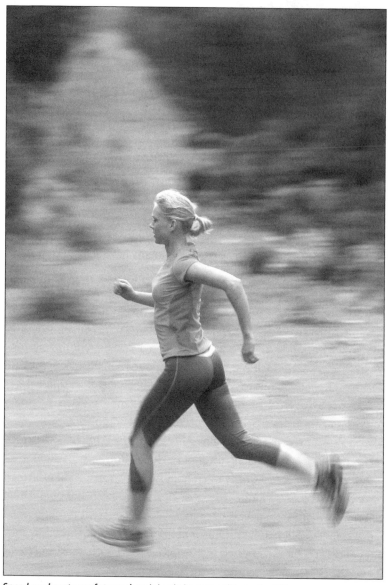

Speed can be a type of strength training in its own right. Stephan/Gripmaster certified trainer, take a resistance training class at a local recreation center or gym, or check out a book or video on weight training.

THE BASICS OF STRENGTH TRAINING

Resistance training, if blended into a trail running regimen, should incorporate at least two sessions per week. But do not work the same muscle group two days in a row. Such back-to-back workouts are counterproductive because it takes approximately forty-eight hours for the body to repair any microtears that occur with resistance training. If you choose to visit the weight room every day, rotate workouts so that you work legs one day and the upper body the next. Some runners who focus on weight training work specific muscle groups one time a week, such as the back on day one, chest and triceps on day two, legs on day three, shoulders and biceps on day four, and so forth.

Be creative and flexible in the gym, and ensure that the weight-training program reinforces rather than detracts from trail running. For example, if a race is coming up on the weekend, avoid doing a hard leg day on Thursday or Friday. Rearrange your resistance training schedule and replace a heavier weight day that would have fallen close to a race with a session that uses body weight for the exercises, such as dips, pullups, pushups, situps, crunches, or leg raises.

Resistance machines, such as Nautilus or Cybex, which isolate specific muscle groups, are easy to use without a spotter and without much experience. Free weights and cables, which draw on a fuller range of muscles, require proper form. They tax the major muscle group worked as well as the supporting muscles. Depending upon the availability of resistance machines or free weights, personal resistance training experience, strength, susceptibility to injury, and your personal goals, you can custom design the perfect routine that strikes a comfortable balance with the equipment at your disposal.

In addition to working on proper form for each exercise, focus on breathing while strength training. Exhale when exerting and inhale when finishing each repetition.

Upon selecting the exercises to include in a resistance routine, decide the correct starting weight, number of repetitions, and sets to be performed for each exercise. A repetition ("rep") is the movement that completes the exercise through the lifting (positive or concentric) and lowering (negative or eccentric) stages. In general, runners need not lift more weight than they are able to complete in at least eight reps without compromising form. It is also important to ensure that the routine selected works opposing muscle groups equally in order to avoid an imbalance that can damage running form and lead to injury.

If you desire to gain substantial strength, perform enough reps to hit the point of "failure," the point at which another rep is not possible without losing proper form. The "pursuit of failure" is an odd concept, but it works in the gym. Sore muscles the next day or two after a challenging resistance day is as satisfying as the need to walk down stairs backward after a race, because those aches are evidence you really pushed yourself.

The number of reps performed to complete an exercise sequence is called a "set." Runners probably don't need to perform more than one or two sets of any exercise. However, if you are determined to build strength and don't mind building up muscle mass, you may opt for an occasional low rep/multiple set day where the focus is on working a particular muscle group.

Weight training usually increases appetite, especially for high-protein foods. Resistance training raises your resting metabolism, so be prepared to eat more if you incorporate resistance training in your training routine.

Are the Weights Making Me Fat?

After lifting for several weeks, you may feel as though you have lost some weight only to step on the scale to discover that the opposite has occurred. Because muscle weighs more than fat, those new to weight training often find that their clothes fit more loosely even though their weight is the same or has increased. Keep overall objectives in perspective: If you feel better, are stronger, and have healthier muscle tone, why be concerned if you have not lost weight?

THE BASIC ROUTINE

Beginning with the upper body, a routine should focus on chest, back, biceps, triceps, and shoulders. If you work the entire upper body in the same session, work larger muscle groups first and the smaller groups last. After warming up with some exercises that use only body weight, such as pullups, pushups, dips, or light stretching, work on pectorals or chest and the latissimus dorsi ("lats"), the triangular back muscles below the shoulders.

Chest and Back

To work the chest, mix and match among pushups, dips, dumbbell press and flies, flat, incline, and decline bench press, chest machines, and cable flies. You may experiment with altering the width separating the placement of your hands on the equipment, but the general rule is to maintain approximately shoulder width. For lats, select and combine pullups, lat pulldowns, seated rows, one-arm rows, back machines, and cable rows.

Shoulders

To work shoulders, perform shoulder presses with barbells, dumbbells, or a shoulder press machine. Also beneficial are straight arm lifts with dumbbells or a cable machine, with elbows locked to isolate the shoulders. Shoulder injuries from lifting are rather common, so be sure to use caution with proper form and light enough weight to avoid any harm. Other exercises for working the upper body include shrugs, upright rows, and reverse flies for trapezius muscles, which lie between the shoulders and neck in the upper back. Strong trapezius muscles are important for trail runners because they are taxed when you hold out your elbows on rugged terrain to maintain lateral balance and quick responsiveness.

Biceps

For biceps, do curls with a curl bar, dumbbells, a machine, or cable. Curls can be performed either standing or seated, with a "preacher" bench or other devices that help isolate biceps. When doing standing curls, be careful not to swing your upper body by throwing the back and/or shoulders. If necessary, wear a weight belt to protect the lower back or lean against a wall or post to prevent swinging.

Triceps

The triceps brachii is the muscle that extends down the back of the arm from shoulder to elbow. There are many ways to work the triceps, and it is a good idea to use different exercises because of the unique makeup and qualities of this "three-headed" muscle. Choose among triceps kick-backs, triceps dips, cable pulldowns, reverse triceps cable curls, and cable or dumbbell pullovers.

The Lower Body Workout

Runners tend to be touchy about weight training for legs. Many feel that just running is sufficient to strengthen the lower body, especially when they run on hilly or mountainous trails. True, running makes legs strong; but resistance training makes them stronger, and stronger legs can translate to faster, better, and usually injury-free running. It is not uncommon for a trail runner to experience significant gain in uphill speed after undergoing a weight training routine for a couple of months. More powerful calves, quadriceps, hamstrings, glutes, and hip flexors help power you up a climb on which you might otherwise have struggled.

The following leg exercises help build lower body strength and can be done with free weights, cables, or machines, depending on what is available and your personal preferences:

- leg extensions

- squats

- hamstring curls or leg flexions

- dead lifts

- calf raises (seated and standing)

- toe raises

- adductor and abductor exercises

- hip flexor or high knee raises

- lunges

Working one leg at a time, at least for a few sets, helps to correct any strength imbalance between your legs. Though more common for road runners, disparity between the strength of hamstrings and quadriceps—generally, when quads are more than twice as strong as hamstrings—can manifest itself in too short a stride. Work the hamstrings at a weight at least half the weight used to work the quads.

Proprioception (or "Wobble") Boards

Another type of leg workout particularly well suited for trail runners is to use proprioception boards or "wobble" boards for strengthening and conditioning the micromuscles that are used for balance. Proprioception is the body's ability to orient itself in space without visual clues. The ability to use your muscle, joint, tendon, and inner ear sensory nerve terminals to adjust posture and positioning through stimuli originating from within the body is not "The Force." It is proprioception.

Proprioception boards are usually made to work both side to side and forward-backward to balance. A common proprioception board is a narrow board that is fastened to a short half-sphere. Stand with one foot or both feet on the board and do exercises such as squats while balancing. This helps to develop the muscles that are crucial to stability, such as ankle support muscles.

Abdominals

A strong and flexible trunk is also quite important in trail running; the abdominal muscles are crucial to posture, back support, and stability, plus they assist in absorbing some pounding on descents. To be a trail runner you need catlike balance, responsiveness, and a strong and limber back to maintain those qualities. Because abdominal muscles support the back, never neglect the stomach when it comes to strength training.

One can work abdominal exercises into lifting routines by weaving situps, crunches, and other simple trunk strengtheners into the mix as short breaks between sets, regardless of whether working on legs or upper body. Trunk exercises include crunches, leg lifts—either with the back on the floor, hanging from arm grips, or on a leg lift stand—incline bench crunches, exercise ball situps, and roman chair back extensions. Various trunk machines and gimmicky anti–love handle exercise accessories are also an option. To work the supporting muscles on the sides of the abdomen (the obliques), you can use a roman chair for side-ups or, when working situps and crunches, raise your head and neck up to one side, then the other.

CHAPTER 6

Stretching for the Trail

Although athletes have focused on flexibility for decades, coaches and trainers have only recently begun to stress the importance of stretching. Stretching used to be something smiling people wearing leotards did in black-and-white television programs while they bounced through what has become an antiquated school of ballistic stretching: "And one . . . two . . . three . . ." Since those days, the art of stretching has changed dramatically, and trail runners may now choose between myriad techniques, including active-isolated stretching, static stretching, and stretching through disciplines such as yoga.

Stretching is fundamental to gaining and sustaining flexibility, which is a crucial element of trail running. By maintaining a regular stretching routine, you are able to help muscles, tendons, and ligaments remain supple to avoid injury. Stretching staves off stiffness and rigidity brought on by training and racing, and increases elasticity and resilience of connective tissues. Stretching also aids in recovery, injury prevention, stride length, strength, and nimbleness on the trail.

The stretching tool kit contains many implements. One type is active movement such as dance, martial arts, or certain types of yoga. This type of stretching is *dynamic* stretching. Another tool is to pose in a position that causes you to feel a stretch and challenges the muscles' reflex to contract. This practice, called *static* stretching, gradually pushes the reflex or contraction point, thereby building flexibility.

Another type of stretching is through the use of training partners, trainers, stretching aids, and a battery of new stretching devices. These tactics not only enable you to expand your stretching routine, but they also provide new ways to remain limber while building strength and developing supporting muscles for improved flexibility and balance while on the run.

There is a great diversity in stretching philosophies, and each school of thought has its own set of guidelines. However, good commonsense rules of stretching should apply to all trail runners. They are as follows:

- **Warm up before stretching.** Warm muscles are less prone to strains (pulls), sprains (tears), or other injuries. Depending on the temperature outside, the place of the warm-up, the particular warm-up exercise, and its intensity, the pre-stretch period should be approximately the time that you would take to cover a flat mile. And do some stretching after the run to prevent post-workout soreness.

- **Use proper form to isolate particular target muscles.** If you are unsure about proper form for a particular type of stretching, take a stretching class at a local health club or recreation center, consult with a personal trainer or coach, or check a book on stretching. Bob Anderson's book, *Stretching*, remains one of the better texts on the subject. Build a repertoire of stretches that addresses your particular needs, and stick to it as a regular part of your training schedule.

- **Don't bounce.** Ballistic stretching (bouncing through a stretch) triggers a reflex that has the effect of tightening muscles. Ballistic stretching may also lead to a strain or other damage caused by bouncing beyond one's natural range of motion. Using a long, sustained static stretch after warming up releases tension that has built up in the area of focus.

- **Breathe into the stretch.** Isolate the muscle that is the goal of a particular stretch by continuing to breathe as you feel slow elongations of the targeted area. Stay relaxed and use slow rhythmical breathing. Hands, feet, shoulders, jaw, and face should not reflect tension.

- **Stretch to the point of "pull" not pain.** According to Anderson, a mild comfortable stretch should result in tension that can be felt without pain. Do not gauge a stretch by how far you can reach; go by feel alone.

- **Pay special attention to all injuries**. In some cases, stretching may make a particular injury worse or prolong recovery. It may be worth consulting an expert before engaging in any stretching routine while injured.

- **When performing a static pose, hold the stretch for as long as thirty seconds and stretch both sides equally.** Anderson recommends that when doing a stretch, you should feel comfortable enough with the tension that it can be held for ten to twenty-five seconds, after which the initial feeling of the stretch should subside or disappear. That kind of stretching reduces muscle tension and maintains flexibility. To increase flexibility, Anderson recommends a "developmental stretch." After an easy stretch to the point where the feeling of tension dissipates, go into the pose again—but go deeper—until increased tension is felt. The stretch should not feel any more intense when held ten to thirty seconds. If it does, ease off to a more comfortable position.

Incorporate the above rules as you customize a stretching routine that fits and appeals to your particular needs.

THE BASIC STRETCHING ROUTINE

Consider incorporating some of the following stretches into your stretching regimen. These suggestions are by no means exhaustive, and it is recommended that additional resources be consulted to select and perfect an appropriate personal stretching routine.

Hamstrings

A modified hurdler's stretch involves sitting with one leg bent and that foot tucked against the inside of the thigh of the extended leg. From that position, lean forward (keeping the back straight) from the hips until tension is felt in the hamstring of the extended leg (see Figure 1). Another hamstring stretch is to lie flat on your back, lift one leg at a 90-degree angle with the other leg bent and its foot on the ground (see Figure 2). A third hamstring stretch is to stand with one leg raised so that the foot rests on a solid object, such as a stool or a rock that is about at knee level. With the standing leg slightly bent, lean forward from the hips, keeping the back straight, and reach for the ankle of the extended leg until stretch is felt in the hamstring of the extended leg.

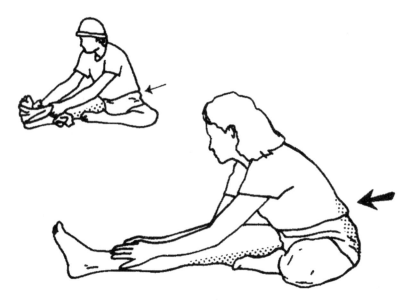

Figure 1. *Straighten your right leg. The sole of your left foot will be resting next to the inside of your straightened leg. Lean slightly forward **from the hips** and stretch the hamstrings of your right leg. Find an easy stretch and relax. If you can't touch your toes comfortably, use a towel to help you stretch. Hold for thirty seconds. Do not lock your knee. Your right quadriceps should be soft and relaxed during the stretch. Keep your right foot upright with the ankle and toes relaxed. Do both legs. Breathe relaxed.*

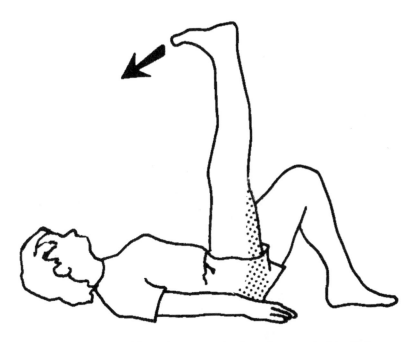

Figure 2. Lie on your back, lift your leg up toward a ninety-degree angle at the thigh joint. Keep the low back flat against the floor during the stretch. Hold stretch for fifteen to twenty seconds. Do both legs.

Iliotibial (IT) Band

The band that stretches from just behind the hip, running down the side of the leg and connecting to the top of the shin, is the IT band. When the IT band tightens, it can cause a flare-up on the side of the knee, resulting in pain. If a runner persists in running with a problematic IT band, it can ultimately seize up like an engine that has run dry of lubrication.

Any one or all of the following stretches can keep the IT band loose and flexible. In a sitting position with both legs stretched in front, cross one leg over the other and cradle the crossed leg in your arms, pulling the shin and foot of the crossed leg toward the chest until stretch is felt in the hip of the bent leg. Or, see Figures 3A and 3B for a two-phase stretch. Or, from a standing position, cross one leg in front of the other and lean forward to touch the toes until tension is felt in the hip of the rear leg. In the same pose, stand more upright and lean into the hip of the rear leg until tension is felt.

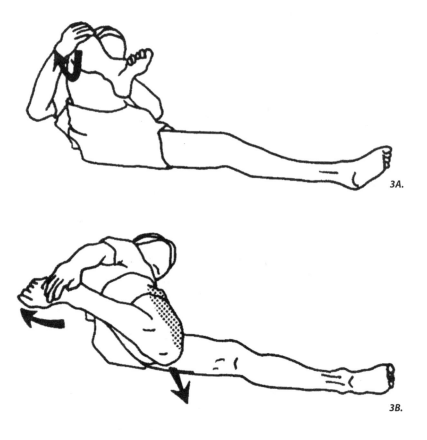

3A.

3B.

Figure 3A. *Lie on your side while holding the front of your lower leg from the outside with your right hand. Circle your leg in front of you, then slightly behind you. As you circle your leg, move your right hand to the top of your right ankle.*

Figure 3B. *Now you should be on your side as in the bottom figure. To stretch the iliotibial band, gently pull your right heel toward your buttocks as you move the inside of your knee downward toward the floor. You should feel a stretch on the outside of your upper leg. Hold for fifteen to twenty seconds. Do both legs.*

Groin and Hips

Because trail runners consistently have to dodge obstacles on the trail, they must employ considerably more lateral motion than do road runners. Sudden movement from side to side can lead to a pull or strain in the groin and hips, unless that area is properly limber. One easy stretch is to sit down and place the soles of both feet against each other a comfortable distance from the groin. Then slowly lean forward from the hips until a comfortable stretch is felt. Increase the tension of the stretch by pulling the heels closer to the body or lowering the knees to the ground by gently pressing elbows downward on the inside of the lower legs—not on the knees (see Figure 4).

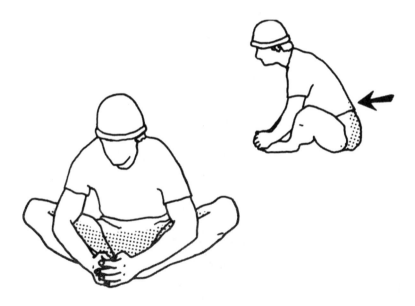

*Figure 4. Put the soles of your feet together with your heels a comfortable distance from your groin. Now, put your hands around your feet and slowly contract your abdominals to assist you in flexing forward until you feel an easy stretch in the groin. Make your movement forward by bending **from the hips** and not from the shoulders. If possible, keep your elbows on the outside of your lower legs for greater stability during the stretch. Hold a comfortable stretch for twenty to thirty seconds.*

Quadriceps

Descending a rocky trail at a fast pace places considerable stress on the quadriceps. A number of stretches can be performed to loosen your quads. One easy stretch is to stand on one foot and bend the other leg backward, reaching back with the opposite hand to hold the foot of the bent leg, lifting the foot to the point where a stretch is felt (see Figure 5). Another stretch—one that should not be performed by those with weak ankles or problem knees—is to kneel on the ground with both knees, feet pointed backward. Lean backward until the quads feel a stretch. Another basic quad exercise that helps to build flexibility is to perform a static squat by slowly bending the knees while keeping the back straight and your weight centered over your pelvis.

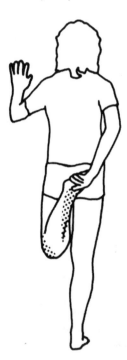

Figure 5. *Opposite hand to opposite foot—quads and knee stretch: Hold top of your left foot (from inside of foot) with your right hand and gently pull, heel moving toward buttocks. The knee bends at a natural angle in this position and creates a good stretch in the knee and quads. Hold for thirty seconds. Do both legs.*

Calves

Nonrunners often chuckle at the sight of runners who, when posed in this stretch, appear to be trying to push over a building or lamppost. This stretch involves standing about an arm's length from a wall, post, tree, rock, or other fixed object and placing both hands against the object. Bend one leg and place your foot on the ground in front of you as the other leg is stretched straight behind, keeping the heel of the straightened leg on the ground with the toes facing forward. Lean into the rear leg until that calf is stretched (see Figure 6).

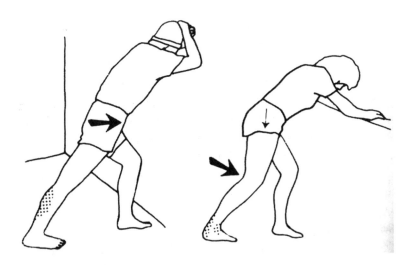

Figure 6. To stretch your calf, stand a little ways from a solid support and lean on it with your forearms, your head resting on your hands. Bend one leg and place your foot on the ground in front of you leaving the other leg straight, behind you. Slowly move your hips forward until you feel a stretch in the calf of your straight leg. Be sure to keep the heel of the foot of the straight leg on the ground and your toes pointed straight ahead. Hold an easy stretch for thirty seconds. Do not bounce. Stretch both legs.

*Next, to stretch the soleus and Achilles tendon, slightly bend the back knee, keeping the foot flat. This gives you a much lower stretch, which is also good for maintaining or regaining ankle flexibility. Hold for fifteen seconds, each leg. This area needs only a **slight** feeling of stretch.*

Devoting substantial time to stretching calves pays off, especially if focus is on the full range of the gastrocnemius muscles. Maintaining calf flexibility is very important for trail runners who tend to run high on their toes or do a lot of hill work. For those limber enough to be able to touch their toes, another way to stretch the calves is to sit on the ground and extend both legs parallel straight in front. Lean forward from the hips with your back straight and hold the toes, pulling them toward the body until a stretch is felt in the calves. If you cannot touch your toes, loop a band or towel around your toes, then pull on it to stretch the calves.

Ankles and Achilles

One of the greatest problem areas for trail runners is weak ankles. Maintaining flexible ankles helps prevent ankle rolls or sprains and enables you to recover from what could be a casualty. Ankle rotations are easy to perform and can be done even while sitting. Lift one foot a few inches off the ground and slowly rotate it through its full range of motion. Rotate it in both directions. To stretch the Achilles tendon, stand with one leg raised so that its heel rests on a solid object that is about at knee level. Lean forward, place both hands under the ball of your raised foot, and gradually pull it toward the body. After feeling the stretch, point the toes toward the ground as far as possible.

Back and Trunk

Trail runners should invest heavily in a limber back and trunk. A tight back or midsection can lead to a nightmare of injuries, terrible running form, and an unhealthy posture. Practicing yoga on a regular basis can lead to a flexible back and relaxed running form. Back and trunk stretches include a standing waist twist where hips are rotated in one direction as you look over your shoulder and hold the stretch, with hands on hips, knees slightly bent, and feet pointed forward. For a standing back extension stretch from the same standing position, place palms just above the hips with fingers pointing down, then slowly push the palms forward and arch the back to create an extension in the lower back, and hold the stretch.

Another easy back and side of hip stretch that releases tension that may build up from running hills or rocky trails is to sit with your right foot resting to the outside of your left knee, then pull your knee across your body toward your opposite shoulder until an easy stretch is felt on the side of the hip. Hold for fifteen seconds (see Figure 7). An additional lower back stretch involves lying on your back with one leg extended flat on the ground. Bend the knee of the other leg and cross it over the extended leg, using the arm on the side of the extended leg to gently pull the bent knee down toward the ground, keeping both shoulders flat until a stretch is felt (see Figure 8).

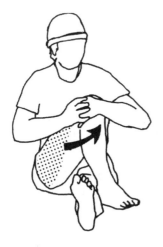

Figure 7. With your right foot resting to the outside of your left knee, pull your knee across your body toward your opposite shoulder until an easy stretch is felt on the side of the hip. Hold for fifteen seconds. Repeat to other side.

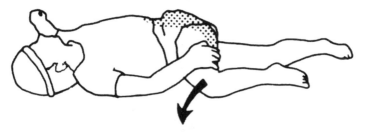

Figure 8. Bend your leg and, with your opposite hand, pull that bent leg up and over your other leg as shown above. Turn your head to look toward the hand of the arm that is straight (head should be resting on the floor). Make sure the back of your shoulders are kept flat on the floor. Now, using your hand on your thigh (resting just above the knee), pull your bent leg down toward the floor until you get the right stretch feeling in your lower back and side of hip. Keep feet and ankles relaxed. Hold a comfortable stretch for thirty seconds, each side.

Upper Body

Trail runners tend to use their arms more than road runners, due to the need for balance and occasional trail touchdowns or scrambling. Because of this, it is important to keep your arms loose. The same goes for the neck and shoulders. Long ascents or descents can cause tension in the upper body. The advantage of most upper body stretches is that they can be done on the fly, providing relief without the need to stop. If you grow tense during a run, try flapping the arms about wildly and jutting the hips around in a very silly display. In addition to laughing at yourself—and encouraging anyone in sight to laugh as well—this odd behavior releases built-up stress and at least temporarily realigns running form into a more relaxed and efficient posture.

To loosen tight shoulders and lower neck tension while not running, incorporate slow-moving "windmills" (shoulder rotations with swinging arms) and exaggerated yawning-type movements in both directions. Rotate your head around in all directions, but be careful in trying this on a run, since it tends to momentarily compromise balance. For a more intense stretch, apply slight pressure on the head with your hands as the head is rotated. For good measure, throw in some shoulder shrugs, lifting the shoulders up toward the ears. To loosen the arms, raise one at a time, folding it at the elbow behind the head while using the other arm to gently apply pressure so that the hand of the bent arm flows down the upper back.

CHAPTER 7

Equipment

If you are a trail runner, then your equipment needs are diverse. Gear must be light and sufficiently performance oriented so as not to inhibit running; yet it must be durable and functional enough to hold up to the rigors of the trail. Given these needs, you are as likely to find proper gear by shopping at an outdoor outfitter as you are by shopping at a running specialty store. Above all, wear what works, functions, and fits—far larger concerns than is fashion.

SHOES

Not long ago, it was enough for you to walk into a store that sold running shoes and tell the salesperson that you liked to run on trails. You were immediately steered to one or, if lucky, two or three styles of shoes appropriate for trail running. Fortunately those days are gone. Now, however, you might be perplexed by the opposite problem: selecting the "right" shoe from among over seventy styles of trail shoes made by nearly twenty manufacturers.

The process of buying trail running shoes varies tremendously from person to person, and is often haphazard. Like finding the perfect life mate, the decision often centers on the right "fit" and the goal of having an enduring relationship. So it is important to shop around, learn from the experience of past selections, and stick with what works.

An informed decision requires answering some probing questions. To help take the mystery out of trail shoe purchases, you can save time and effort by categorizing yourself as a certain "type" of trail runner. Although the process of trail runner classification is hardly scientific, it is a bit more precise than shoe shopping with a tarot card reader or astrologer and can help you narrow the decision to a few different styles, at which point you can apply the Cinderella technique of going with the best fit and feel.

Which of the following characteristics best describe you as a trail runner: stable or unstable, heavy or light, nimble or clumsy, hot or cold, cheap or lavish, ultra rugged, versatile, or fashionable? Keep in mind that just as these adjectives are not necessarily mutually exclusive, a single shoe style might not apply to a single runner type. Indeed, you may want multiple pairs of trail shoes to use for different types of runs. It is not uncommon for trail running devotees to fill a closet with racing shoes, training shoes, mixed (road and trail) shoes, and maybe a pair of semi-retired shoes for ugly conditions or lawn and garden work.

The following checklist should help you determine what type of trail runner you are for purposes of selecting at least one pair of appropriate trail shoes:

- Are you injury prone?

- Do you need special support or stability built into the running shoes?

- What is more important: fashion or function?

- On what types of terrain will the shoes be used?

- How many miles are expected from the shoes before retirement?

- Are either breathability or waterproofness of uppers important?

- How much do you want to spend?

- For runs of what distance will the shoes be worn?

- Is it important that the shoes be designed for women?

- Are your feet sensitive to bone bruises?

- Do your feet have an unusual size or shape?

- Is shoe weight an important factor?

- Is the shoe's low-profile "trail feel" important?

Answers to these questions help you—or at least a running store clerk—to make more informed trail shoe purchasing decisions. Once armed with this information, you will also find it easier to replace a favorite shoe style when the manufacturer discontinues or completely changes the model after only one season.

Those prone to injury should seek the help of a healing arts practitioner or a sports trainer skilled in analyzing gait, stride, or other factors that may explain the source of a specific injury. That information will help determine the best shoe to promote alignment without sacrificing performance or comfort.

A treadmill test that allows a runner to run barefoot and then wear different shoes while being videotaped helps analyze gait, detect certain running problems, and determine how various shoe styles correct or exacerbate any biomechanical idiosyncrasies. Some specialty running shoe stores provide treadmill tests for free to their customers. Physical therapists and other sports medicine professionals also offer comprehensive analyses of running form. Going the professional route may be expensive, but the information provided from these trained experts is very valuable, especially if it prevents an injury.

Scott Jurek, multiple winner of the Western States 100, provides such analysis at the Foot Zone in Seattle, Washington. Patrons of that running store benefit from Jurek's dual status as a physical therapist and accomplished trail runner. If you are fortunate enough to live near a specialty running store that provides treadmill analysis, tactfully inquire as to the qualifications of the salesperson providing the analysis so as to determine how much credence to give to the salesperson's advice.

Shoe Construction

To begin the trail shoe selection process, one needs to understand a bit about the anatomy of a running shoe and what distinguishes trail shoes from road shoes.

Tread

From the bottom up, a trail shoe usually has a more aggressive tread, or outsole, and deeper lugs than a road shoe, and some have a reverse or "directional" tread pattern for downhill control. The outsole provides traction and is usually made of a durable carbon rubber and/or other compounds to enhance traction, stabilize or smooth out the "ride," control motion, and increase longevity.

Midsole

The next level up, the "midsole," is the heart and soul of a trail shoe. The midsole is usually made of ethylene vinyl acetate (EVA) or polyurethane (PU) to provide most of the cushioning, support, and stability. The decision of when to retire a trail shoe should depend on the compression of the midsole. Those shoes that feature relatively firm midsoles tend to provide a more rigid ride and are more popular with ultrarunners because that type of shoe maintains its integrity and proves very durable over the long haul.

A trail shoe's midsole composition also determines its profile, or how low to the ground the foot sits in the shoe. A low profile offers a greater sense of contact with or "feel" for the trail. And although a low profile enhances agility, it provides less protection from bone bruises. On the other hand, a more substantial midsole offers greater cushioning but limits a runner's ability to feel the trail—performing more like an RV than a sports car.

Many manufacturers integrate multiple materials into the midsole to help give the shoe more stability or motion control for runners that supinate (a pronounced outward roll of the ankle) or overpronate (a severe inward roll of the ankle). These materials have different densities, known in the shoe manufacturing trade as "durometers," that are controlled to determine the shoe's flex point and overall flexibility. A denser material that is used in the arch of the shoe to reduce pronation is called a "medial post." Some shoes also feature hard heel counters and other rear foot stabilizers to control overpronation.

Some trail shoes feature reinforcements, such as a fabric weave or a carbon plate, in the midsole to protect the foot, especially the metatarsal or ball of the foot, from bone bruises. Shoe companies also integrate various gel capsules, air compartments, or other cushioning devices into midsoles. While some of these shock-absorbing devices work well for road shoes, they are often little more than gimmicks when it comes to trail shoes; in many cases they detract from the performance or stability of the shoe while adding substantial cost.

Another aspect of a trail shoe is what is known as the shoe's "last" or shape. There are three primary types of lasts: straight or board lasted, curved or slip lasted, and a combination of the two, which is aptly called a combination last. Although the last has more to do with how the shoe is manufactured, its importance to runners is that the last determines the shape of the foot bed—either straight or curved. Although runners frequently favor one shape over the other, the choice of a last really comes down to a subjective "feel" test of overall fit and performance. Recognizing the difference between the shape of a man's and a woman's foot, many shoe manufacturers have begun building women's shoes that are not merely smaller versions of men's shoes, but are actually built on a woman's last.

Sock Liner and Upper

Above the midsole, the next layer is the sock liner or insole, which may be removed to accommodate orthotics, arch supports, or other corrective devices. Topping off the entire shoe is the upper, which secures the foot to the midsole. Trail shoes are usually constructed with one or a combination of mesh, leather, synthetic leather, or a waterproof breathable fabric.

Trail shoe uppers benefit from being a bit more rugged than their road counterparts, but not to the extent that the shoe is overbuilt and heavy. Because of the increased abrasion from the trail, trail shoe uppers often feature reinforcements, such as hefty toe bumpers that protect against stubbed toes. Trail shoe uppers should and usually do provide more lateral support than road shoes. Much of this support and stability comes from the heel counter, which holds the foot in place over the foot bed. Some trail shoes offer additional lateral stability, especially in the heel, through a higher-collared upper. Like classic basketball shoes, these trail shoes cover the ankle joint and are popular among runners prone to ankle rolls.

The lacing systems of trail shoes allow runners to choose from a variety of fastening options that adjust the fit for comfort, pressure distribution, and stability. Many trail shoes also feature more flexible laces that reduce pressure on the instep and tend to stay tied when wet. Nylon laces have an aggravating ability to loosen themselves, especially when wet.

The Deciding Factors

Knowing the terrain on which the trail shoes are most likely to be used helps in selecting the appropriate tread, midsole, and upper materials. For example, a "hybrid" (trail/road) shoe is best for mixed runs on paved roads and trails. Some runners prefer road shoes to trail shoes because they do not like the extra weight that is often associated with trail shoes that are built with thick midsoles, beefy toe bumpers, overlay protection on the uppers, and treads that are so aggressive they resemble equipment made by a mountain bike tire manufacturer. If you log most of your miles on pavement and only a small fraction on trails, a road shoe may be the best choice, especially if you are particularly fond of the smoothness and lightweight qualities offered by a road shoe. Alternatively, you might consider a hybrid shoe that for all intents and purposes is a road shoe with a beefier outsole, toe bumper, and earthier colors.

If you spend most of your time on singletrack, sand, scree, ice, mud, gravel, rock, and other challenging off-road surfaces, you should look for trail shoes with aggressive tread patterns. Keep in mind that softer outsole materials effectively grip rocky surfaces but wear more quickly than harder carbon rubber. Trail shoes often have two or three durometers of outsole materials placed in strategic parts of the tread to maximize traction and durability.

Pricing and Durability

Another consideration is the number of miles that you can reasonably expect from the shoes before they must be retired, coupled with how much you are willing to spend on the footwear purchase. Discounts and clearance sales aside, the price for a decent pair of trail shoes will vary from around $60 to $130. Though somewhat ironic, it is frequently the case that lower-priced trail shoes have longer lives than the more expensive models. This is explained by the fact that the more expensive styles often feature relatively complex support systems and/or are constructed with more cushioned midsoles, which are prone to breaking down or compacting. Not only do those who need or desire more cushioning have to pay a steeper price for each pampering purchase, but they also must make more frequent purchases.

The relative stiffness of the midsole is the most important consideration in selecting a shoe that will endure over the miles. The stiffer the midsole, the longer the shoe will retain its original cushioning. When shopping for a trail shoe, you can test midsole stiffness by flexing a shoe in your hands and bending the toe back at the ball of the foot. The relative resistance is a good gauge of the relative stiffness.

Mileage Covered

It is helpful to anticipate the usual distance over which the shoes will be worn. For shorter distances, it is fine to go with lighter shoes that have very aggressive outsoles and minimal support or cushioning. If you plan to run longer distances, you will want shoes that give plenty of support, breathe well, and have midsoles that remain consistent over different types of surfaces and under different weather conditions. One thing to keep in mind is that feet almost inevitably expand after hours of running, especially at higher elevations. Many experienced ultrarunners, for example, buy shoes at least a half size larger than normal to accommodate this common occurrence.

Weather Conditions

You should also consider the likely weather conditions of your runs and your individual need for ventilation, waterproofing, or warmth. For example, if you are likely to be running in wet climes, through morning dew, or in mud, slush, puddles, or other wetness, you may want to consider a shoe that either shields out water or that is sufficiently breathable to enable moisture to be quickly squeegeed away. Trail shoes with waterproof liners or barriers are likely to retain moisture or condensation that builds up inside. Many trail runners opt for shoes that have mesh uppers, and wear them with wool socks so that water exits the shoe as easily as it entered. Wool socks better maintain a moderate temperature and prevent blisters.

Similarly, if you have hot feet, then you need shoes that breathe through effective ventilation. Those individuals should look for shoes with lighter mesh uppers and no or minimal leather or synthetic overlays. They might also consider running "sandals," which have open uppers and use strapping systems to secure the foot to the midsole.

Some General Tips for Buying Running Shoes

- Look at the wear and tear of your old, "spent" shoes. Are the soles worn in certain parts and not in others? Wear patterns provide evidence of overpronation or supination.

- Observe your wet footprints left after a shower, bath, or swim and compare your prints with others. This will help you determine your relative arch height and forefoot width.

- Knowing your particular "foot notes," you are better prepared to go to a specialty running store, catalog, or online vendor and ask an expert salesperson for a recommendation.

- It is best to go to a running specialty store where a foot specialist can perform a gait analysis with a videotaped treadmill or other test.

- When shopping for trail shoes, wear the same kind of socks that you use when you run. Similarly, if you use orthotics you should bring the devices to ensure shoes fit once the orthotic is inserted. It is best to shop immediately or soon after you run, when your feet are most likely to be swollen.

- Be wary of buying a new model or style of shoe from a catalog or Web site. Just because you liked a brand of shoe does not mean you will be happy with another model or style from the same manufacturer. Likewise, just because you enjoy a particular shoe model does not guarantee that the next iteration with the same model name will fit or perform in a similar manner. Shoe manufacturers are always tweaking their lines in an effort to better the product, and all too often those "improvements" leave the runner with a shoe that goes by the same name but has an entirely different feel, fit, or performance.

Biomechanics

Those with special needs due to biomechanics, sensitivities, or genetics must be more selective when purchasing trail shoes. That includes runners who need additional cushioning or have odd-size or abnormally shaped feet. Many shoes on the market offer increased support or stability and some incorporate additional cushioning. A handful of trail shoe manufacturers strive to accommodate certain types of feet, and some produce trail shoes in different widths.

Another strategy that may appeal to trail runners with idiosyncratic feet is to try socks of different thickness or amounts of padding built into them. Some sock manufacturers have woven new materials into the foot beds, while others use wool with knit-in padding. If you use orthotics, you must make sure that the shoes fit them, given the particular last.

In the gender arena, for many years women had to purchase shoes that were designed primarily for men, with "the other sex" a mere afterthought resulting only in varied shoe colors or reduced sizing. Fortunately, manufacturers have acknowledged this deficiency and are now catering to female trail runners with specially engineered women's shoes. Numerous women's trail shoes on the market are manufactured on a woman's last, so before purchasing check to see how that affects fit and comfort.

Style

Trail runners driven primarily by the looks of their shoes should get a life, be banished from the trails, and hit the roads. Oops, did we say that? Although appearance should only be a final consideration, to completely ignore its importance would be unrealistic. For those trail runners who really care about aesthetics, check out one of a number of Web sites that enable customers to design their own shoes while online. Customers can select colors, logos, and other cosmetic qualities and have the shoes made to order in a couple of weeks for a price that is competitive with most ready-made shoes on the shelves.

Weight

Finally, if you are stable and agile, especially if you are fast enough to care about shoe weight, you will want to avoid the overbuilt, tanklike trail shoes that many manufacturers make with the thought that it is better to doze *through* trails rather than run *with* the trail. Too many manufacturers view trail runners as essentially hikers who just go a little faster, and accordingly, they produce trail shoes that are more akin to hiking boots than running shoes. Fortunately, a few companies make more nimble, lightweight running shoes for the trails that will appeal to lighter, more agile runners.

Make Your Trail Shoes Last Longer

The best way to prolong the life of trail shoes is to have several pairs and rotate them so that one pair is never used for more than a couple of consecutive runs without getting a rest. Using an old beat-up pair on days when the weather is particularly "sucky" also extends the life of newer shoes that you would rather not expose to brutal conditions. Like allowing the body to have recovery days, giving shoes some time off allows the midsole materials—the parts that usually break down the fastest—to decompress between runs.

It is a good idea to wash shoes by wiping them down to remove caked mud. Remove the insole inserts from the foot bed and insert wadded up newspaper in the foot bed while the shoes dry at room temperature. If the shoes were soaked, it may be necessary to replace the newspaper once or twice.

It is best to allow shoes to dry slowly. That way they will be less likely to delaminate. Do not run them through the washing machine or dryer or put them in the oven, which can damage the midsole material. Keep wet shoes out of the microwave! Finally, reserve favorite trail shoes for the activity for which they are made. Do not wear them to work or for walking or hiking because that compresses and stresses them in ways that are not conducive to running, plus such activities break them down prematurely.

APPAREL

A favorite saying among outdoor sporting goods retailers is that "there is no such thing as bad weather, only bad gear." Unlike road runners, who tend to wear apparel made by shoe manufacturers or "fast forward" types of apparel companies that make clothes designed for triathletes, cyclists, and more urban athletes, trail runners tend to buy clothing designed for the outdoors or mountain type. When it comes to dress, trail runners are as likely to wear clothes made for skiers, climbers, kayakers, or mountain bikers as they are to wear runners' attire. Focus on the durability and functionality of a garment, paying careful attention to the performance of the fabric and placement of closures, hoods, pockets, and venting. In general, trail runners are not particularly concerned about the style of their clothing.

With the advent of modern fabrics, improvements to old materials, and technological breakthroughs that help moderate body temperature and maintain dryness from both inside perspiration and outside precipitation, the weather is no longer an excuse for not hitting the trail. Dressing properly—especially for those who run trails under extreme weather conditions—has become a science of its own. You should choose garments with the same care with which you approach training and racing. An error in selecting clothing can ruin what would otherwise be a pleasant trail adventure and may have far more deleterious effects.

Seasoned trail running veterans are often victors over younger, faster athletes simply because less experienced competitors fail to dress appropriately. The wrong mix of clothes can result in overheating and dehydration or, conversely, to chilled muscles and even hypothermia. Running when too warm forces the body to perform in a suboptimal microclimate. That inefficiency leads to poor performance. Fortunately, with today's high-tech fabrics, even the greenest trail runner finds it easy to enjoy their experiences in varying weather conditions. Although modern textiles have come a long way, some of the old basics still rule. Wool is still one of the best all-around fabrics because of its wicking, thermal, antimicrobial, and resilient qualities, especially in its new washable and itch-free versions.

Layering

Layering has been popular, as well as wise, and even fashionable at times. (Recall when the *The Preppy Handbook* was a national best seller in the early 1980s, when it was all the rage to traipse about wearing a turtleneck, button-up, and sweater—in pink and green, no less.) Layering has always presented a practical approach to coping with variable weather conditions and/or differing exertion levels.

Layering can be broken into three primary categories: base (against the skin), mid (also known as the insulation, thermal, or performance layer), and outer (shell). While the following discussion is divided into these three layers, keep in mind that several manufacturers, mostly in the outdoor industry as opposed to the running industry, have designed some excellent pieces of apparel that blur the layering distinctions by incorporating two or even all three layers into a single garment. There are many excellent all-in-one versatile items that wick moisture like a base layer, provide fleece-like insulation, and feature microfiber windproof and water-repellent outer layers to make them ideal single items to wear or carry when uncertain of weather.

Marino Giacometti, president of the International Skyrunning Federation, advises trail runners who train and race at high elevations to wear tights and a long-sleeve synthetic top. For longer training or racing runs, Giacometti finds it indispensable to wear or at least carry a lightweight, windproof vest or jacket, gloves, headband, sunglasses, and a hydration system. "The temperature and conditions can change rapidly at altitude and mountains are more exposed to wind, so be prepared," he says.

Base Layer

Worn next to your skin, base layers tend to be soft and are primarily designed to wick moisture from the skin so that it can be evaporated through outer layers, while providing some warmth. Cotton, once very popular among runners as a base layer, has gone the way of the dodo bird. Cotton is not recommended as a base layer fabric because it retains moisture, does not breathe well, and becomes abrasive to skin when wet. In contrast, modern merino wool—which does not itch—is an ideal base layer material because it maintains dryness with an all-natural body temperature regulation and moisture control system that works so well that sheep use it year-round! Wool breathes well, absorbs and wicks moisture, and is resistant to fungus. Newer performance wools can be run through the washing machine and dryer without shrinking, felting, or otherwise changing shape.

The importance of an effective base layer must not be overlooked: A trail runner can wear the most advanced shell on the market, but it will be worthless if he or she is soaking wet on the inside. Ideally, a base layer maintains a sufficiently warm or cool temperature so that the runner is neither shivering nor sweating. By avoiding overheating, a runner will release less moisture, which helps to maintain better hydration and performance. Most technical synthetic base layer fabrics are known as "hydrophobic," which means that they repel moisture instead of absorbing it. Polyester, nylon, and polypropylene are the most common hydrophobic fabrics.

Be considerate of your trail running partners by choosing a base layer that is resistant to body odor, which is caused by bacteria, ammonia, and denatured proteins that are components of sweat. Different manufacturers fight odor-causing microbes by weaving bacteria-killing silver strands into the base layer fabric, or by using a coconut fiber that neutralizes odor-producing agents or a chemical antimicrobial in or on the fabric. Trail runners with sensitive skin or environmental agendas should be aware that some of the antimicrobial chemical coatings are the same chemicals used in pesticides. If those chemicals are problematic for you, look for base layers that are hypoallergenic.

Base layers should be somewhat formfitting or tight. Some moisture wicking fabrics work best if they are snug against the skin. That contact allows them to wick moisture at an early stage. Some fabrics are even able to transport moisture while it is in the vapor state. Base layers should fit well with the trail runner's particular body type, and if chafing is a concern, select pieces that use flat-seam construction. When selecting a top, be sure to choose the neck style that is most comfortable from among crew, mock, turtleneck, half zip, or full-length zip.

Similarly, purchase an appropriate top from tank, sleeveless, short-sleeve, or long-sleeve styles. When selecting a jog bra, women should consider a fabric that wicks, stretches to form fit, and supports without binding or rubbing under the arms or breasts. Jog bras that come in a variety of cup sizes and chest measurements provide a better, snugger, more supportive fit than bras that are sized by just small, medium, large, and extra large. The styles are as varied as a woman's figure, so choose a jog bra based on comfort and fit.

Finally, another quality of base layers, especially if they are likely to be worn by themselves, is the level of sun protection that the fabric offers. Mesh or loosely knit fabrics do not block many harmful rays, so if that is all that is worn, consider applying waterproof (read: "sweat-proof") sunscreen or block under the base layer. More densely woven base layers do a much better job of blocking sun rays. But those particularly sensitive to the sun should check the sun-blocking characteristics of their trail running wardrobe.

Midlayer

The second layer, known as the mid, thermal, or performance layer, is a continuation of the base layer in managing moisture. However, the midlayer also provides thermal insulation. Midlayer fabrics work with the base layer to transfer moisture to the outer layer and are often made of the same hydrophobic materials but with a more spacious weave. Fleece, especially microfiber fleece, works well as a midlayer because it has moisture transfer qualities, boasts a high warmth-to-weight ratio, and is not bulky. Some thermal layer fabrics use quilted weaves or other patterns that incorporate air pockets for increased warmth.

Outerwear

Finding an ideal outer layer or shell presents the puzzle of balancing or achieving both breathability and water resistance. With the goal of keeping you warm and dry by resisting or blocking the elements, such as wind, rain, or snow, the shell must also allow perspiration to escape through vents and technical features in the fabric. Except under extreme conditions, totally waterproof fabrics are overkill and even undesirable for trail runners. Waterproof materials tend to add bulk, inflexibility, and expense and especially reduce breathability in the garment. A storm-proof outer layer sounds great if you expect to confront freezing rain, but if the jacket and pants do not breathe well, you quickly become as wet from sweat on the inside as you would have had you chosen shells that lacked any water-resistant properties.

In most conditions you will be served best by wearing microfiber outer layers that allow molecules of body-temperature vapor to escape while being windproof and water *resistant,* rather than waterproof. Micro-fiber garments are often less expensive, weigh less, pack smaller, and are more pliant and therefore less noisy than their waterproof counterparts. Some manufacturers have applied laminates or encapsulating processes to enhance the windproof qualities and water-resisting performance of microfiber apparel.

Important qualities that distinguish functional trail running shells from those that are better used for other outdoor recreation include the presence and optimum placement of venting systems, pockets, hoods, cuffs, closures, lining, and abrasion-resistant panels. When consider-ing the purchase of a jacket with all the bells and whistles, think about whether the weight and cost of each zippered, snapped, Velcroed, or cord-locked opening is necessary. For example, "pit zips" have become relatively common in modern jackets, but they serve little function because they are placed directly under the arm, where it is difficult for air to circulate. Some manufacturers have noted that fact and moved the zippered vents toward the chest to enable air to enter the shell and vent the wearer's core.

Decide what style of shell—pullover "shirt," full-zip jacket, or vest—is best. Also consider the costs and benefits of such features as self-storage pockets, and the integration of other fabrics in various panels, such as fleece, stretch material, breathable, wicking, or mesh back sections. If night running in the presence of motor vehicles is part of your regime, reflective taping is a worthwhile feature. Finally, try on the jacket to check the collar height and look for the presence of a fleece chin cover to pro-vide protection from exposure to or abrasion from cold zipper pulls.

Running Shorts and Tights

When it comes to running shorts, you will primarily want to look for the best style or cut. Running shorts that are meant for the trail tend to be designed with a fuller cut and often feature some pockets and perhaps a belt. Like trail shoes, trail shorts are all too often overbuilt and bulky. While some lightweight fabrics that are used for road running shorts may not endure the rigors of trail running, most suffice quite well, unless repeatedly subject to scrambling, glissading, or butt sliding. Shorts usually feature integrated wicking briefs. Women should steer clear of a nylon brief and opt, in this one instance, for cotton instead.

When it comes to running in the cold, trail runners can keep their legs warm by choosing between tights and "loose tights" (also called "relaxed fit pants" or "track pants"), all of which are made from wicking base layer fabrics with Lycra, Spandex, or other resilient materials blended in to make them soft, flexible, and quite warm. When it is really cold, double-layer tights, tights with windproof panels, or wind pants over tights usually keep the legs adequately warm. Whether wearing shorts, tights, or pants, consider wearing an underlayer of Lycra, Spandex, wind briefs, or wind shorts that feature strategically placed front microfiber panels to protect the more sensitive parts of the anatomy from chilling winds. As multisport speedster Darrin Eisman puts it: "For guys, the cold weather brings another 'little' concern . . . a cold windy day can lead to penile frostbite. And while I have not heard of any cases that involved amputation, I have definitely scared myself on a few winter runs." Wearing fuller-cut undershorts as a base layer under tights or running shorts will also reduce inner-thigh chafe.

Socks

Trail runners—normally a mellow lot—can become quite animated and adamant when it comes to socks and their preferences in material, collar height, and even color. Choice in thickness may depend on shoe fit. As far as color is concerned, those in the white sock camp should know that they fight a losing battle. White trail socks do not stay white and usually morph to a faded version of the color of the soil on a favorite trail.

Regardless of those preferences, the most important qualities in choosing socks for trail running are temperature regulation, moisture management, cushioning, and protection from blisters. Some trail runners prefer thin synthetic socks that have minimal cushioning and offer a better trail "feel." Others find that thicker wool socks maintain a comfortable foot temperature in varying weather, in wet conditions, or on trail runs with water crossings. Those concerned about cushioning may opt for socks that are constructed with various weave patterns in different zones of the foot bed to enhance cushioning and comfort. Many trail runners run in trail shoes that feature relatively firm midsoles and temper that rigidity with cushioned socks.

Head and Hands

You should think twice before setting out on a jaunt without a hat or cap atop your head. Caps, especially those with bills, protect the scalp and eyes from sun and reduce the chances of overheating. Many caps are made out of moisture-wicking materials and some feature mesh sides for venting heat. Some hats made specifically for blocking the sun have been constructed of a fabric with a high SPF rating and feature draped flaps that shield the neck from the sun's rays.

Given that approximately half the body's heat escapes through the head, hats are the single-most important item of apparel for maintaining warmth. As a means of adjusting for a more comfortable temperature, many hats can be rolled up or down to expose or cover ears. If you will be running in extreme cold, look for hats that are made with fleece, wind-blocking materials, wool, or a combination of fabrics that preserve warmth yet wick away perspiration under a variety of foul-weather conditions. When the temperature is particularly frigid or if the windchill factor makes exposure and frostbite a real danger, it may be necessary to run with a face covering, neck gaiter, or balaclava to protect skin.

Mittens are much warmer than gloves, and if manual dexterity is not a concern, mittens are probably a better choice for colder climes. Besides, given the fortunate lack of rude and inconsiderate drivers to curse on trails, there is no need for that middle finger. Some trail runners wear bicycling or weightlifting gloves with padded palms to protect their hands from falls or when scrambling.

Gloves and mittens are made of a variety of different fabrics and vary in thickness. Some are made of moisture-wicking, windproof, or water-proof fabrics, while others feature high-tech materials that are either integrated into or coat glove or mitten linings to maintain a comfort-able temperature. If the hand temperature rises above the engineered comfort zone or "target" temperature, the material absorbs the heat and stores it for subsequent release should the hands cool below the target temperature. As a final consideration, if the back of mittens or gloves is likely to be used as a nose wipe, make sure that fabric is soft.

ACCESSORIES

Eyewear

Running eyewear has progressed enormously in the last decade to the point where sunglasses are now functional as well as looking pretty cool. Because you will be constantly using your eyes to scope out your next steps and enjoy the awesome views, your eyes are very valuable assets—ones worth preserving. With lighter frames, full protection from harmful ultraviolet rays, and lenses that shield from insects, dirt, and shrubbery, modern glasses are worth wearing.

Today's eyewear also tends to be versatile, sporting features such as adjustable bridges and temples and interchangeable or photochromatic lenses to accommodate changes in brightness. Some sports glasses have venting features that prevent lenses from fogging. Other attributes to consider include rubberized bridges to prevent slipping and straight or wraparound frames that relieve temple pressure.

When shopping for trail running eyewear, look for lenses that offer full UV protection and also look for lens shades that work well in variable lighting, especially if glasses will be worn when running in and out of forest shadows. Sports eyewear prices range dramatically. Make sure the glasses have the features that are most desirable before buying a pair of cheap gas station glasses or investing a week's wages in some designer shades.

Electronics

In general, trail runners are not big consumers of modern technological devices, at least when compared to road runners, mountain bikers, or triathletes (aka "tri-geeks"). Nonetheless, certain gadgets can add to the trail running experience if used discreetly. A *cell phone* carried in a hydration pack can be a lifesaver in the event of an emergency. But one used to call a broker from a mountaintop to find out how the market is performing is likely to be a real buzzkill to others on the trail. Then again, relying on a cell phone can be a problem because signals are often unavailable in remote areas. *Two-way radios* are also another option for added safety.

Watches used to be devices that told the time of day and perhaps the date. Now, however, a "wrist-top computer" can tell the barometric pressure, weather trends, altitude, heart rate, direction, global positioning, ascent and descent rate, distance run, pace, and splits and compare all of that information against logs from previous excursions. Whether knowing any of that data is desirable is a subjective question, but some of it can be quite helpful. Trail runners are now able to explore new terrain with fewer worries of getting hopelessly lost or being hit by an unexpected storm. Nor will they have an excuse for being late.

The use of a *digital compass, altimeter,* or *GPS* (Global Positioning System) may enhance the trail running experience, especially when a run covers unfamiliar ground or isolated terrain. If alone and hopelessly lost or seriously incapacitated, a GPS can locate your position anywhere on Earth within about a couple of yards; that information and a cell phone could save a life. The combination of GPS and communication devices can also facilitate a more enjoyable and stress-free run among a group of runners who like to go at different paces by enabling coordination of a successful rendezvous.

Heart rate monitors, discussed in Chapters 3 and 4, are helpful for those who pursue certain fitness and training goals, especially trail runners who tend to overtrain. Depending on the level of technical sophistication, monitors can be programmed to sound an alarm when the measured heart rate exceeds or drops below a preset training zone. Some monitors record and store the session's heart rate data, and for those who are fascinated with analyzing numbers, some heart rate monitors are capable of downloading information to a personal computer to keep an accurate log and chart fitness developments. Devices that use foot-mounted *motion sensors* can also provide workout information as to distance covered, pace, and splits.

For wrist-mounted electronic devices, consider wearing the unit on an adjustable nylon or elastic band, perhaps with a Velcro closure. Such bands allow for a broad range of adjustability and can fit over gloves or mittens. They also tend to be more comfortable in varying temperatures. Consider the conditions under which the electronic devices are likely to be used and make sure they are waterproof and have adequate battery power.

Flashlights and headlamps are important devices for trail runners who run in the dark, especially ultradistance runners who are likely to race or train without sunlight. Many types of flashlights and headlamps are on the market, so weigh anticipated needs against the different attributes of various light sources. A flashlight provides precise directional focus, but usually requires one hand to hold it. In contrast, headlamps free the hands, but some runners find the light angle makes it difficult to discern trail obstacles because it is always shining from above.

Flashlights and headlamps come in different weights, brightnesses, and with a variety of light sources, such as halogen, fluorescent, LED (light-emitting diodes), and conventional tungsten lightbulbs. These different types of lights vary in brightness, energy efficiency, durability, and cost. Some units allow for adjustability in brightness and intensity of focus, while others come with rechargeable battery packs and water-resistant or waterproof qualities.

Packs, Hydration Systems, Gel Flasks, and Water Filters

Given the paucity of water fountains, spigots, or other conveniences on the typical trail, it is wise to carry liquid and nutritional reserves. Depending on the temperature, projected length of run, availability of potable water, and the particular hydration and nutritional needs of an individual trail runner, it may be necessary to carry substantial quantities of drink and food on a long trail excursion.

For shorter outings, you will likely be able to get by without any liquids or food. But as temperatures rise and the distance of a run lengthens, you will, at a minimum, need to carry a 16- or 20-ounce bottle of water or sports drink. Depending on preference, bottles may be carried in hand, either by simply gripping the bottle or with the assistance of a strap that fastens the bottle around the back of the hand, or in a lumbar or "fanny" pack. Modern lumbar packs that are designed to distribute weight evenly throughout the lumbar region often feature straight or angled pouches for bottles and separate pockets for food, clothing, and accessories. Some lumbar packs also include "gel holsters" to carry a flask that holds up to five packs of sports gel for easy consumption and relief from sticky fingers or the need to pack out trash.

For longer runs, especially on trails that do not come in contact with sources of potable water, a hydration pack or multibottle carrier is probably necessary. Hydration packs have become common accessories in the evolving world of endurance sports because of their convenience and functionality. They work through a bladder or reservoir, delivery tube or hose, and a bite valve that allow trail runners to carry substantial quantities of fluid that are evenly distributed on the body and consumed with hands-free ease. Hydration packs range in size and carrying capacity and come in the form of backpacks, lumbar packs, and sports vests. Many hydration packs offer additional volume and storage pouches for food, clothing, and other trail necessities. Certain bite valves are easier to use than others, and some bladders are more difficult to clean or keep free of bacteria, mold, mildew, and fungus. Others come with antimicrobial compounds, and some feature in-line water filters.

When running on trails that cross many water sources, whether they be streams, creeks, rivers, ponds, lakes, or merely large puddles, feel free to relieve yourself of substantial weight by carrying water filters and only a single water bottle. Make sure the filter removes such evils as Cryptosporidium, *Giardia, E-coli,* volatile organic compounds, and other threatening substances that are common to the local water. Note, however, that water filters do not protect against viruses. It may be necessary to use a combination of iodine tablets with a filter to ensure that water is safe for consumption.

When considering a pack that is suitable for a trail run, one of the most important attributes to look for is a snug fit that carries the load firmly against the shoulders, small of the back, or lumbar region. The ideal pack should have just enough volume to carry the bare necessities of fluids, food, clothing, accessories, and emergency or safety gear. It should be stable and feature a compression system that can allow for a larger load to shrink as the run progresses (and fluids and food are consumed) without becoming a floppy or abrasive mess. Other aspects of well-designed running packs include multiple compartments; ease of adjustability; nonflapping straps, clasps, and attachments; durability of materials and stitching; ease of access through strategically placed pockets and zippers; hydrophobic next-to-body fabrics; venting systems; expandability through hinged pockets; bungee cords; and daisy chains.

MISCELLANEOUS GEAR

Poles

With the growth in adventure racing, Skyracing, and Nordic walking, sightings of runners who use ski poles on their runs has increased. Poles are not just for dry-land ski training anymore. Runners use them to help redistribute the workload from their legs to the upper body, especially on ascents. Poles also help one's balance. They should be light, sturdy, and easy to carry when not in use. If the poles have baskets, they should be minimal in size in order to avoid entanglements and reduce awkwardness in use. While sharp points make the poles excellent spears for charging beasts, they also do a fine job on one's own foot.

Gaiters

Consider wearing low-cut gaiters, even when there is no snow around. Gaiters prevent gravel, scree, sand, stones, or dirt from penetrating the ankle collar of shoes, thus relieving a buildup of trail debris at the bottom of your shoes or the annoyance of having to stop to remove the offending substance from shoe and sock. Some trail shoes are now designed with gaiter attachments or snug-fitting ankle collars to prevent any intrusion of debris.

First Aid and Emergency Tools

For safety, consider carrying a first-aid kit, snakebite kit, or some basic backcountry safety items like a lighter, about 20 feet of lightweight rope, and a Swiss Army knife, Leatherman, or other multipurpose tool. Maps are very useful, too. It might also be wise to pack a whistle or mace to repel uninvited advances, whether animal or human. Consider bringing duct tape—the universal solution, panacea, and fix-all that works in a pinch as a makeshift gaiter, blister preventer or mender, cut patcher, splint, tourniquet, garment rip stopper, etc. In sum, if a trail emergency can't be remedied with duct tape, it's time to worry! Dermabond or other glues for skin cuts are also quite helpful.

Crampons

If you live in colder climes, you may need some added traction before braving icy trails. Running crampons come in several varieties, and depending on the extensiveness of ice, depth of snow, and prevalence of rocks and other hard surfaces under and surrounding the ice, you will want to select crampons with teeth of the appropriate aggressiveness and materials. Some crampons have relatively shallow teeth that are made with softer substances, like rubber or plastic, while others feature long fanglike claws made of metal alloys. Ski poles are also helpful when ascending icy climbs.

Running Strollers

Parents and others who care for children and wish to share with them the pleasures of trail running will be pleased to know that some modern all-terrain running strollers are built to handle trails at a running pace. These strollers are sturdy enough to withstand the trials of the trail and are also designed to keep little passengers safe and sound. Most running strollers have strong brakes, "parent leashes" to prevent runaway casualties, multi-point child harness systems, and antiroll protection, while some even offer suspension to cushion the ride for the young occupants.

Dog Accessories

For those who run with canine companions, some of the leashes on the market make life a lot easier. There are "hands-free" leashes that are worn around the waist and attach to the dog's collar via quick-release mechanisms for safety and convenience. Other leashes are made from elastic shock cord to allow some play without excessive slack, a real convenience when trails are rocky or otherwise require quick maneuvers that may not coincide with movements of the dog.

Another handy item is a leash pack that conveniently slides over a leash in which to carry "poop bags," both empty and full. Collapsible lightweight bowls pack onto a leash or in a fanny pack to make it easy to keep four-legged trail runners well hydrated and fed on the run. And don't think the convenience of energy bars is restricted to human consumers. Several brands of energy bars for canines are available in an array of flavors that are made of healthy, calorie-packed ingredients with nutritional attributes aplenty.

Bryon Powell's Equipment Tips

Bryon Powell, author of iRunFar.com, *shares some additional equipment tips:*

While at its roots trail running is the simplest of sports requiring nothing more than an open route and the will to cover it, the right gear can make your next trail run easier, safer, and more enjoyable. The right gear is particularly useful in keeping you hydrated, keeping you on course, and keeping you on the trail after dark.

Hydration

In summer proper hydration is crucial, and it remains important year-round. The simplest means of providing hydration on the trail is carrying a bottle or two filled with water or your favorite electrolyte beverage. To make things easier, a number of companies sell "handhelds," which are essentially straps that wrap around the top and bottom of a water bottle while hugging your hand between the bottle and the strap. Most handhelds have a small pocket for carrying a key, ID, and an energy gel or two.

If you prefer to have both hands free while running, try a waist-belt bottle pack. Bottle packs are available in one- or two-bottle varieties and have pockets ranging from minimal to almost a liter. You may need to test a few varieties before finding a bottle pack that doesn't bounce. To save money, go for a run with a friend's bottle pack. There's little use in testing a bottle pack in a store, as it will feel much different when holding full water bottles.

For runs on which you will need more water, food, or gear, try a hydration pack. Choose a hydration pack that will meet your needs for hydration (bladders range from 50 to 100 ounces) and gear (storage space goes from near nothing to 30-plus liters). An exterior bungee is a great way to get a wider range of uses from one pack. A bungee allows you to purchase a pack with a smaller internal compartment while still being able to stash a jacket or hat easily for changing weather conditions.

For any hydration system in which you'll be carrying a key, make sure it has a key hook. In cold weather, use an insulated hydration system that will keep your beverage flowing throughout your entire run!

Navigation

One of the easiest ways to get into trouble on the trail is to not know where you are. To safely navigate the trails, one can rely on time-tested methods. Learned trail knowledge, a map (with or without compass), and trail markers are hard-to-beat methods if you are comfortable with them.

There are also a few pieces of technology that can help you find your way around the trails when using traditional navigation methods. For instance, when you combine something as simple as a watch with some knowledge of how fast you travel over various terrains, you can estimate how far you have traveled down the trail. Although far from 100 percent accurate, foot pod accelerometers are another way to estimate how far you have traveled down a trail. If you are carrying a topographical map on the trails, the altimeter in an adventure watch can help you pin down where you are on a trail or how far you still have to climb to the next pass.

While a few intrepid souls have been using larger GPS devices since the late 1990s, newer wrist-top GPS devices offer an easy, convenient way to navigate the trails. Before a run, you can upload a GPS route from previous runs (your own or others) or from software such as National Geographic's Trails Illustrated Explorer. If, on the other hand, you prefer to head out to explore the trails on your own, some wrist-top GPS devices have a "back to start" feature that can guide you home should you get turned around. Be aware that GPS devices may lose signal and, therefore, be useless in tight canyons or under dense canopy. A dead battery can also leave you wandering on the trail.

While not used as much for navigation as safety, you and your loved ones now have the option for a sky-high safety blanket in the form of devices like the SPOT Satellite Messenger. Basic SPOT service allows a trail runner to send loved ones an "I'm OK" message, a help request, or, if necessary, a request for emergency services. All of these messages include GPS coordinates. An additional SPOT service updates a user's location every ten minutes, allowing those at home to keep track of a runner's progress on the trail.

Lighting

Perhaps no other type of trail running gear has come so far in the past decade as lighting systems. Long gone are the days of needing to carry a spare incandescent bulb in case one burned out or broke during a fall. These days, nearly indestructible LED-based lights are the standard. In addition, LED brightness and battery life are improving at an incredible rate.

Most trail runners prefer using an LED headlamp, because with a headlamp the light automatically follows where you are looking, while also leaving your hands free. Any of the brand-name 3-ounce LED headlamps at your local outdoor store are well suited for trail running. Choose one that fits well (not too much pressure, but doesn't bounce either) and that suits your preference of longer battery life versus brighter maximum output.

Some trail runners prefer adding a second light source lower to the ground to highlight obstacles on the trail. Most of the time this second light is an LED flashlight that is often brighter than a standard headlamp. A flashlight is not only useful for casting shadows from rocks and roots, but also for spotting trail blazes or anything else that may require additional light. Other runners prefer to wear a second headlamp around their waist, which provides the shadow-casting benefit of a flashlight while still leaving the hands free.

At least one company now offers an LED lighting system that attaches to the shoulder straps of a pack and another system that attaches directly to a waist belt. These systems provide the same benefits of a headlamp worn around the waist while being easier to get on and off.

CHAPTER 8

Nutrition On and Off the Trail

Diet and nutrition are two of the most important and undervalued components of a well-rounded athlete's training plan. According to Lisa Dorfman, director of sports nutrition and performance for the University of Miami and author of *The Reunion Diet* (Sunrise River Press, 2010), a trail runner's daily caloric needs are in direct proportion to gender, size (height/weight), metabolism, and fitness level. Then consider the amount of energy expended through daily activities (i.e., walking the dog, cleaning the house), training intensity, duration, and environmental conditions such as temperature and elevation. The overall daily goal is to consume a carbohydrate-rich diet to replenish the body's limited muscle and liver glycogen stores and to consume the balance of calories from lean protein, fruits and vegetables, lowfat dairy or substitutes, and essential fats.

Because training regimens vary widely among trail runners, so do their nutritional requirements. This chapter concentrates on the basics of food as fuel, vitamins and minerals, and, most important, key fueling time periods: before, during, and after a workout, training run, or race. Maintaining a critical balance among these three time frames is what every athlete strives for to help achieve the highest level of performance and recovery. However, it is useful to first understand the basic elements that make up a healthy athlete's diet.

CARBOHYDRATES

Carbohydrates are the preferred fuel burned by muscles during exercise and should comprise about 5 to 7 grams of carbohydrate/kg of body weight for easy-to-moderate running days and 7 to 12 grams of carbohydrate/kg of body weight per day for "hard" training sessions. Total calorie intake should match calorie expenditure; thus protein and fat can be adjusted to meet total daily calorie needs based on fluctuations of carbohydrate intake. Carbohydrate fuel spares protein in muscle, preventing excessive damage and breakdown, and helps the runner use fat as a long-term energy source. Endurance training and intense repetitive sessions are dependent on adequate blood sugar levels to maintain energy in order to access stored sugar or fats. Without enough daily carbohydrates, performance and recovery suffer. Your body has about ninety minutes worth of carbohydrate fuel in the tank, so choose simple sugars to refuel during the run because they enter your bloodstream more quickly and give you immediate energy, whereas complex carbohydrates take longer to digest and are more a part of your day-to-day intake.

Complex carbohydrate sources are in foods like whole grain pasta, rice, bread, and cereals; whole grain pancakes, waffles, and oatmeal; and other grains (i.e., quinoa, barley) and starchy vegetables (i.e., potatoes, sweet potatoes, peas, corn, etc). All are rich in vitamins, minerals, and fiber as well as plant compounds called phytonutrients, which aid in recovery and performance. "Discretionary calories" from simple carbohydrates come from foods containing simple sugars such as sport drinks/shakes, bars, and gels, and are excellent for extending training duration. There's always room for a little dark chocolate and a sweet treat—just keep it around 10 percent of your daily calories. (Do the math: That's 280 calories for someone consuming 2,800 calories.)

PROTEIN

Protein is important for running because it's the glue that holds the runner together. Protein assists in recovery by preventing muscle breakdown, contracts and relaxes muscles, and builds ligaments and tendons that hold muscles and support bone. Protein is also needed for building hormones like insulin, which regulates blood sugar, maintaining the thyroid for metabolism, and supporting the immune system. Protein slows digestion and in turn helps you feel full for longer periods of time. Try to include a little protein at each meal and/or snack if you will be going longer than three to four hours without a scheduled meal. Without adequate dietary protein, you can fall apart through injury and illness. While protein is not the primary fuel for the actual run, it is part of the support system. And while protein can provide energy to runners in times when carbohydrate and fat are depleted, it's not ideal since protein is required for more important duties such as keeping the immune, metabolic, digestive, and structural systems healthy. High-quality proteins from chicken, fish, turkey, red meat, eggs, and soy provide all the essential amino acids—the building blocks of protein that must be supplied by the diet in the right amounts.

For runners who train four to five times a week for forty-five to sixty minutes, all you need is about 1.2 grams of protein/kg per day and up to 1.7 grams/kg if you're adding strength and cross training to the mix. For someone who weighs 150 pounds (68 kilograms), that's 81 grams of protein per day at the lower recommendation. It's easier than you think to consume enough protein: A typical 6-ounce chicken breast is equal to 42 grams, and if you drink two cups of milk daily, that equals 16 grams. Add a slice of lowfat cheese (8 grams) and ¼ cup nuts (6 grams) and you've just about met your daily needs. It was once theorized that vegetarians needed to "combine" all their proteins at each meal to make a "complete" protein; however, as long as you consume a variety of vegetable proteins throughout the day, your body will get all the complementary amino acids just as it would with meat sources. Substitute the animal portion for a combination of beans, peas, nut butters, soy (i.e., tofu, edamame, tempeh, protein bars), and deli or frozen "meat" alternatives, or add protein shakes with soy, whey, or other plants high in protein such as hemp. Vegetarians who avoid all animal products may fall short of some minerals such as iron and zinc depending on the type of foods consumed. If you have concerns, check with your doctor or a registered dietitian to obtain a computer nutrient analysis of your diet to see if you are getting the right amounts.

FAT

A certain amount of dietary fat is essential to absorb the fat soluble vitamins A, D, E, and K. Other fats called omega-3 fatty acids, which come from flax or grains (ALA-Omega-3) or fish and algae sources (DHA/EPA-Omega-3), can act as anti-inflammatory agents. Fat is used as energy during long, slow, and less intense training, helping to conserve muscle glycogen so it can be used during latter portions of a workout. The calories in fat (9 kcal/gm) are more than double of carbohydrates or protein (4 kcal/gm), so eating excessive amounts in food can add extra weight in no time. According to Dorfman, about 30 percent or less of an athlete's total daily caloric intake should come from dietary fats, especially unsaturated fats, which include omega-3 fatty acids for adequate healing and recovery. For most runners this translates to approximately 60 to 70 grams of fat at 25 percent of total calories based on 2,200 to 2,800 calories per day. You may need more or less depending on your calorie requirements. The best unsaturated fat choices include liquid oils such as olive or canola, "light" butter spreads without trans fats or partially hydrogenated oils, ground flax, fish/fish oil, soybeans, olives, avocados, and nuts like almonds, walnuts, or pecans. Select lean meat and consume poultry without the skin.

VITAMINS AND MINERALS

Vitamins and minerals don't have calories like carbohydrates, protein, and fat, but they do help the body use food as fuel and impact every aspect of the runner's health and performance. The two categories of vitamins are fat soluble (A, D, E, and K) and water soluble, such as the B vitamins—thiamine, riboflavin, niacin, pyridoxine, folic acid, pantothenic acid, vitamin B-12—and vitamin C (ascorbic acid). Fat soluble vitamins are stored in the body, so there is less risk of depletion although daily intakes are important as well as adequate fat ingestion for proper absorption. Water soluble vitamins are not stored in the body and therefore must be supplied almost daily to maintain appropriate levels.

Although minerals constitute just 5 percent of body weight, they are essential to cell function. They control the flow of liquids in cell membranes and capillaries, and they regulate nerve tissue and muscle response. Minerals are the essential building materials for blood, nerve cells, muscle, tissue, bones, and teeth, which combine in various ways to form structures of the body and regulate body processes. Magnesium, phosphorous, potassium, sodium, calcium, zinc, iron, and chloride are essential minerals. Food sources include whole grains and fruits, lowfat dairy, red meats, beans, and fortified grains for iron and seafood, nuts, and grains for zinc.

SUPPLEMENTATION

Experts agree that additional vitamins and minerals for performance are unnecessary unless you are deficient in a given nutrient. If runners meet their daily calorie needs, then vitamin and mineral requirements will also be satisfied. Although many runners are well nourished, sometimes life gets in the way. Training, work schedules, low-quality meals and snacks, and lower-calorie diets due to body weight and appearance concerns may lead to a vitamin or mineral deficiency.

Since nutrients can be lost through sweat and vigorous training, a good multiple vitamin/mineral supplement is an inexpensive insurance policy against vitamin depletion. According to Suzanne Girard-Eberle, MS, RD, and author of *Endurance Sports Nutrition,* "Taking a multivitamin/ mineral supplement does just that, it supplements a diet composed of mostly healthful choices." But do not expect a multivitamin to compensate for poor daily eating habits.

The vitamins and minerals of concern to runners include folic acid, the B vitamins, vitamin C, calcium, potassium, magnesium, iron, and zinc. Vegetarians have additional needs to replace iron and vitamin B-12 since it is found primarily in animal products. Runners training early season or for marathon-plus distances may need more of several B vitamins because they are involved in energy production. Katie Mazzia, MS, RD, CDE, clinical dietitian at Vail Valley Medical Center, advises athletes to be aware of the total amount of supplementation ingested on a daily basis through fortified bars or beverages, powders, pills, multivitamin/mineral capsules, energy drinks, etc. Large amounts of one vitamin or mineral may cancel out or decrease absorption of another, and some prescription drugs may interact with vitamin, mineral, and herbal supplements. There is a potential risk of toxicity, and all runners should check with their health care providers if multiple supplements are used, especially more iron than that provided in a general multivitamin/mineral supplement.

When buying a multivitamin/mineral supplement, look at the "Nutrition Facts" label and limit it to approximately 100 percent of the daily value (DV). This amount is generally regarded as safe; however, excess amounts of several vitamins may contribute to serious health problems. Tolerable upper limits (UL) have been established for many vitamins, and runners need to understand that more is not always better. A helpful Web site is www.usp.org/USPVerified.

Female runners who do not consume three servings a day of calcium-rich foods may benefit from a calcium and folic acid supplement (all women of childbearing age should take 400 micrograms of folic acid daily to prevent certain birth defects). Also of special note is Vitamin D: Those living in the upper hemispheres, wearing sunscreen, and limiting food intake of Vitamin D may need to supplement up to an additional 400 IU per day. The maximum UL (upper limit) advised is 2,000 IU.

There are many other vitamin, herbal, and homeopathic aids that claim to enhance performance. It's important to know that ingredients are often not standardized; some contain banned substances not stated or may have side effects and interact with prescription medication. Aside from being costly, most are not harmful and may have more of a psychological vs. physical effect; it's wise to seek additional guidance with supplementation through a registered dietitian or pharmacist. Reference this Web site: www.quackwatch.com.

HYDRATION

Proper hydration helps to prevent weakened muscle contractions. Every ounce of glycogen in muscles requires 3 ounces of water stored alongside. Fluids are provided through food (especially fruit), water, electrolyte drinks, tea, coffee, milk, or milk substitutes. Sport drinks can help to replenish electrolytes along with muscle and liver glycogen to prevent fluid and carbohydrate depletion. Studies show that electrolytes and carbohydrates likely enhance absorption of fluids and flavored beverages aid in increased consumption.

As soon as the run starts, fluids start to empty out of your system through expiration (breathing) and sweat. During moderate activity such as a short run of thirty minutes, you may lose 13 to 20 ounces of fluid and up to 33 or more ounces for heavier activity lasting sixty to ninety minutes. The longer you run the more fluid your body needs. The goal is not to replace 100 percent of fluids lost, but rather to prevent any more than 1 percent dehydration so performance is not impaired. For example, a 150 pound person at 1 percent dehydration would weigh

148.5 pounds after a run. Any more than this and the body will start to feel the effects of fluid loss. To prevent dehydration: (1) Drink fluids throughout the day, (2) Hydrate two to three hours before physical activity with approximately 16 to 20 ounces of fluid, and (3) Drink during and after workouts.

Weighing in before and after workouts can help gauge fluid losses and determine how much fluid is needed post-run. Measuring your weight seasonally will give you guidelines to work with under all conditions. Weigh yourself without clothes before and after a run. If you gained weight, you drank too much. If you lost more than 1 percent of your body weight, you drank too little. Staying hydrated is a 24/7 job.

WHAT TO EAT BEFORE A RUN

A pre-workout meal should consist of mostly carbohydrate-rich foods and beverages, with a moderate amount of protein (less than 10 grams) and a small amount of fat (less than 5 grams). Eat your last meal at least two to four hours prior to a run so the body has enough time to digest the food and prepare itself to use stored fuel throughout your run from muscle, liver, and body fat. If you have eaten a meal and are running in less than two hours, use the principles above—just keep it to about 200 to 300 calories.

Pre-run and race meals vary for every athlete. Some athletes are too nervous to eat solid food, so that's where endurance drinks and energy bars can be helpful. The key is not to eat anything different from what you normally eat during training. Race day is not the time to experiment with food.

If you run first thing in the morning, be sure to hydrate with water or a low-sugar sports drink that will settle in your stomach, and carry additional food and water determined by the length of the run. Even a small amount of mostly carbohydrate food (100 to 200 calories) can improve energy levels after a full night of fasting.

Since fats and oils leave the stomach slowly, they are not suggested as a base for a pre-workout diet. In fact, fat loading before exercise is unnecessary, because even thin runners have sufficient fat stored as body fat for use during exercise.

WHAT TO EAT DURING A RUN

For training or racing that lasts more than sixty minutes, it's essential to keep fueling your muscles with carbohydrates. Endurance running depletes your body stores of carbohydrates, which must be replaced to prevent "bonking." Try to eat at regular intervals from the start of your run or competition and don't wait until you feel tired. The duration and intensity of a trail run, along with the temperature and environmental conditions that will be encountered during the activity, are all factors in determining the nutritional and hydration needs for a run.

Carbohydrates, not fat, are the body's most limited fuel and are the preferred fuel for the brain and nervous system. Even very lean runners have ample fat stores. Carbohydrates are also an efficient fuel for muscles, especially the more intense the pace—the faster you go the more you burn. In addition, the body cannot effectively burn fat for fuel unless sufficient carbohydrates exist to be broken down and drive the body's energy systems. Consuming enough carbohydrates also means the body won't have to resort to using its protein stores (the muscles) as fuel.

In general, runners who perform best are those who eat and drink consistently according to a plan and maintain an even and adequate caloric intake. Liquid carbohydrates are easier to digest and enter the bloodstream quickest; however, solid food can also provide a huge mental boost and stave off hunger pains while on the trail. In training, experiment with different types of drinks and foods so the selection is more varied, and be aware that when the intensity of running increases your body may only tolerate liquid calories. It doesn't work to run for three or four hours and then try to back-load the calories—you'll never be able to eat enough or keep it down.

The late exercise physiologist Ed Burke, PhD, author of *Optimal Muscle Recovery*, reported that those who plan runs under one hour, depending on the temperature and environment, may not need to take any food with them, only water. For runs lasting over one hour, fluids and carbohydrates in a combination of sports drinks, energy bars, water, and gels are necessary to maintain hydration and blood/glucose levels. Depending on particular taste and stomach tolerance, pick the sports drink that works best. Powdered sports drinks are convenient because they provide carbohydrates, fluid, and electrolytes all in one and can easily be carried in a fanny pack to mix with water along the route.

Studies show that carbohydrates from more than one source (i.e., glucose, fructose, maltodextrin, sucrose) allow you to absorb more calories from those carbohydrates, which staves off fatigue. Look for at least two or more sources on the ingredient list of sports drinks or gels. Excessive amounts of sugar from these products may cause cramping and diarrhea while running due to stomach sensitivities to fructose and/or amount of fluids consumed. Aim for 25 to 60 grams of carbohydrate per hour. Individual tolerance may vary and more calories may be needed depending on the event.

For runs lasting more than two hours, stick to low-fat carbohydrates to maintain muscle/glycogen levels and avoid hypoglycemia (low blood sugar). The higher the intensity level, the sooner the effects of muscle glycogen depletion is realized. When running at altitude or on a technical trail, reaction times are critical; hence it is crucial to maintain blood sugar levels in those venues. The ability of carbohydrates to be absorbed into the muscles at the necessary rate depends on intensity, training level, weight, duration, and type of carbohydrates.

As time spent on the trail increases, include other well-tolerated solid foods such as energy bars, cookies, watermelon, bananas, oranges, peanut butter sandwiches, turkey, cooked potatoes, as well as liquid carbohydrate beverages. The longer the run, the more chance the body has to break down these more complex foods that contain varying amounts of carbohydrates, protein, and fat, and use the energy they provide.

Tips from the Trail

Getting in and out of aid stations is a priority for the competitive endurance runner or those not wanting to add more time to their race. Don't underestimate the many uses of 8- to 10-ounce gel flasks. They're not just for gels! Fill them with ramen-type noodles, dilute two to three gels per flask with water, add coffee, add diluted instant mashed potatoes, or make a paste of calories with a concentrated powder or one to two scoops of a recovery drink. In the winter, add a very warm sports drink to a hydration system or insulated water bottle and add hand warmers to the hydration pack where the flow nozzle is to prevent freezing—all brilliant ideas from high-performance runners who realize the importance of calories on the run.

Should an athlete satisfy cravings during a run? Girard-Eberle suggests balancing what the body needs with what is available and stays down. Bonking is an indication that the athlete is running on mere fumes. The brain is shutting the body down so no further damage occurs. In this case, quick-acting carbohydrate-rich foods, such as fruit juice, soda, or sugary candy, are the only options to stabilize the body's blood sugar level. Once an athlete has bonked, special attention must be given to fuel needs during the rest of the run or race. Carbohydrate-rich items, such as sports drinks and gels, fruit/diluted fruit juice, soda, and candy (gumdrops, jelly beans, etc.) are easily absorbed and readily available for use as fuel during exercise. The best energy bars and gels are the ones that work well with and taste good to the individual. Find the best bar and gel through experimentation during training and stick with it for racing. During longer runs, it's wise to have a couple of flavors to switch between to avoid "flavor fatigue."

HYDRATING DURING EXERCISE

Water is an essential nutrient for all runners. The amount required for a trail run depends primarily on perspiration rate, environmental conditions, intensity, and to a lesser extent fluid tolerance level and fitness of the athlete. This makes proper hydration a very individual experience. Performance will suffer even with minimal dehydration, and too much loss may lead to heat cramps, muscle spasms, or heat stroke. The best way to determine hydration levels is to assess your day-to-day hydration level and then translate this information to the trail and a water bottle.

Usually, athletes require about 16 to 32 ounces of fluid per hour; however, this range is only an estimate, and runners must keep in mind the many factors mentioned above. It's nearly impossible to keep up 100 percent with fluid losses, and as little as 1 to 2 percent dehydration (i.e., 3 pounds for a 150-pound person) starts to affect an athlete's performance, resulting in a loss of endurance, strength, and the ability to run at the desired intensity. Drinking too much or too little during exercise can be dangerous and diminish performance.

During activity, how much fluid should an athlete drink? Experts agree that the answer is to start early and often. To prevent dehydration and its ill effects, don't wait until you are thirsty to drink; start sipping fluids at least twenty minutes into your run. The goal is to forestall dehydration rather than trying to reverse it later. Two hours before a trail run, drink between 16 to 20 ounces of water and then refill about fifteen minutes before your run with 8 ounces—especially when the weather is hot and humid. Consume 4 to 8 ounces every fifteen minutes and replace losses post-exercise. According to Katie Mazzia, long runs greater than sixty minutes require a sports drink with about 100 to 200 milligrams of sodium and about 14 grams of carbohydrate per 8-ounce serving; look at the "Nutrition Facts" label on the package and adjust accordingly. Even though you may lose up to 1,000 milligrams of sodium an hour, the goal is to replace about 200 to 500 milligrams of sodium per hour, which can be obtained through a sports drink, gel, or sodium pill; this is of great importance in the marathon and ultra distances. If you do prefer plain water and obtain your carbohydrates from food or lower-sodium gels, you can take sodium capsules (i.e., Salt Stick, S-caps) to replace your sodium. Remember, if you dilute your sports drink, you will dilute the sodium and carbohydrates, and your body will absorb fluids better at smaller intervals versus a large 8-ounce gulp all at once.

Drink Early and Often, Especially on Longer Runs

Sodium is an electrolyte that is lost via sweat in much larger amounts than potassium; therefore it must be replaced during long running events to prevent hyponatremia and allow for optimal fluid absorption.

Be advised that drinking only water during long workouts or races lasting three or more hours can deplete blood sodium levels and result in hyponatremia. This is the most common electrolyte disorder and a potentially life-threatening condition if gone untreated. Excessive sweating, nausea, fatigue, confusion, and even seizures can indicate a hyponatremic condition. Hyponatremia can be avoided during activity by regulating fluid intake, replacing lost sodium and potassium with a sports drink or food, and carefully monitoring perspiration and urination output. When hyponatremia is severe and asymptomatic, restricting water intake usually is safe and adequate, although some experts advocate administration of hypertonic saline.

Risks for dehydration are warm climate, hot gym, long exercise duration, and more than one workout a day. Fortunately, athletes can train themselves to drink more, and at the right points during the run. Since exercise intensity is one factor that determines what empties from the stomach, try to drink on downhill sections where intensity is reduced, thereby allowing more blood to enter the stomach. However, it may prove difficult to drink when descending technical trails, especially during a race.

Under the best conditions it takes twenty minutes to get fluids into the stomach and intestines. If a race requires you to exceed your anaerobic threshold, it may take forty minutes because less blood is going to the stomach. A hydration system such as a hip-mounted unit with flasks, a lumbar or fanny pack, a hand-carried water bottle, or a hydration pack with a bladder or reservoir can help facilitate fluid intake. It helps to train and race with the same system to see what works best for you.

REFUELING AFTER A RUN

In addition to the need to restore the body's fluid balance, muscle glycogen stores need to be replenished. Many runners wait too long to resume eating and drinking following a run. The first thirty to sixty minutes following exercise is crucial to rehydration and recovering glycogen stores.

Because glycogen is so vital, replenishing liver and muscle stores is an important part of recovery from intense exercise. The speed with which the body synthesizes glycogen determines the amount that can ultimately be stored. How fast these stores are replenished determines how quickly an athlete will be ready to compete again or train at peak capacity.

Insulin, a hormone released by the pancreas, increases the transport of glucose into the muscles and stimulates glycogen synthesis. Insulin enables the body to increase its energy stores at an enhanced rate. A narrow window of time exists during which the glycogen replenishment process is most efficient. If glycogen stores are not replenished between workouts, the body may begin to break down muscle tissue to get the protein it needs for energy.

After a trail run, ingest approximately 1 to 1.5 grams of carbohydrate/kg of body weight every hour until a meal is consumed. Fluids with carbohydrates are sometimes easier to get down since appetites are generally diminished right after a trail run. Controversy exists whether protein following a run can enhance absorption of carbohydrates in the recovery phase, but many think recovery sports drinks or bars with protein consumed in the amount of 20 grams or less within the first forty minutes following a run can enhance carbohydrate glycogen recovery.

Girard-Eberle suggests that athletes balance post-exercise carbohydrates and protein according to the optimum recovery ratio, which is 1 gram of protein for every 4 grams of carbohydrates. This balance enhances the insulin response without adversely affecting gastric emptying and rehydration. Again, avoiding dehydration and chronic glycogen depletion is critical for successful future training and racing. Within ninety minutes to two hours following a run, ingest a mixed solid meal with carbohydrates, protein, and fat, for instance a grilled chicken breast with rice, vegetables, and fruit, or a bowl of cereal with 100 percent fruit juice, two eggs and toast, or a baked potato with black beans, salsa, and cheese.

The longer you wait to eat, the more limited the muscle rejuvenation. Mazzia states: "Although there may be times where an athlete will 'train low' in carbohydrates for a few days to push through the fatigue, this should be the exception rather than the rule. Most runners who complain of fatigue have not recovered nutritionally. Eating five or six smaller meals during the day as opposed to two or three large meals maintains blood sugar levels within a narrower range. Optimal muscle recovery is a basic training component in maintaining top physical performance."

Carbohydrate and fluid needs during recovery

Recovery Duration	Carbohydrates (g/kg body weight)	Fluid Replacement (% of body weight lost)
24 hours	8–10 g/kg for the day	Drink enough to maintain body weight
4 hours	1 g/kg each hour	150%
2 hours	1 g/kg each hour	150%
Daily training	5–7g/kg up to 12 g/kg	Drink enough to maintain body weight

SOME FAVORITE FOODS OF TRAIL RUNNERS

Many trail runners surveyed for this book enjoy real food during races and long training efforts in addition to and sometimes instead of energy bars and gels. The following examples illustrate the diversity and creativity of the trail runner's palate. The authors do not necessarily endorse these food choices, but we realize the idiosyncratic nature of trail running gastronomy.

Dave Dunham, who has logged more than 106,000 miles over the past thirty years—many of which have been on trails—has a usual pre-race meal of a plain bagel and coffee at least two hours prior to the race. If the race is less than 10 miles, he doesn't eat anything during the run, and for longer races, he takes a GU or Hammer Gel thirty minutes before the start of the race and every thirty minutes during the race. He has been known to enjoy a Coke and sometimes gumdrops, if the race is marathon distance or longer.

At mile 17 of her last marathon, Wendy Duncan had a friend hand her a piece of cheesecake—her favorite. Duncan recalls, "It was super high in calories, easy to swallow, and gave me a boost before hitting the wall. In fact I even ran a PR! At my next race I'll be indulging at mile 17 again."

Paul Sullivan takes little boxes of raisins on his trail runs. "They're just the right amount to put between my cheek and gums. And, like chewing tobacco (which I don't chew), I can suck on the raisins for quite a while, giving me a consistent, even release of quick carbohydrate."

Paul Charteris likes to put some Nutella and almond butter together in a soft pita. "The extra fat is great for long distance running."

For super long efforts, the value of a Spam sandwich was suggested to Ladd McClain by a coworker and Ironman finisher. "At a time when you can't imagine another gooey gel or energy bar, the seductive aroma of salty pork is quite appetizing—and physiologically I think it has considerable merit. You're low on potassium and salts, and protein requirements are rising as you continue to break down muscle tissue."

After her uncle suffered from hyponatremia during the 1998 Pikes Peak Ascent, Christa Lloyd was careful to consider her fluid and sodium intake during her first Ascent race. "I tried to think about what I could eat along the way that contained lots of sodium. My grandmother offered a solution that I loved: I brought along a little baggie of baby dill pickles. They tasted great during those last few miles!"

High school cross-country coach and former Road Runners Club of America (RRCA) president Carl Sniffen has spent many of his summer vacations running on the mountain trails of Colorado and New Mexico. He says, "There is nothing better than a Bit-O-Honey and diluted Gatorade. The Bit-O-Honey doesn't break apart, and it fills me up for a while. Tootsie Rolls are also tasty and keep their shape in a waist pack. Power-Bars are okay, but not as good as the Bit-O-Honey and Tootsie Rolls."

Jim Nichols has completed the Crow Pass Crossing 26-miler in the Chugach Mountains of Alaska, and has finished the grueling Mount Marathon in Seward, Alaska, multiple times. During his trail runs, Nichols chooses whole food when he can, often taking peanut butter and jelly sandwiches on his runs instead of energy bars.

Roger Sajak, father of two, takes some of his kids' Fruit Roll-Ups and Gummi Bears on long trail runs, eating the first after about one hour. "I don't have to chew them, which is great because chewing and trail running is a hazard, since I can chomp on my tongue accidentally if I hit a slump in the trail or a rock. Gummi Bears, like Fruit Roll-Ups, are soft and dissolve slowly in my mouth, lasting about ten minutes. With the dry air in Colorado, the slow dissolving helps keep my mouth from drying out.

On occasion, I drop a few Life Savers into my water bottle. They slosh around during the run and dissolve after about thirty minutes, giving the water a faint fruit flavor complete with sugar to reduce the fatigue of a long run."

Michelle Blessing, member of the 1995 U.S. Mountain Running Team and former USA Triathlon Olympic coach, craves Slim Jims during her long, hard efforts because they taste great, are easy to get down, are high in sodium, and have protein, fat, and carbohydrates. She also believes in taking in caffeine on long efforts and for that she uses caffeinated gels. If she uses gels, she is careful to consume water so that the carbohydrate of the gel is diluted and more readily absorbed. And for Blessing, drinking a sports drink along with a Slim Jim can completely turn back a rapidly approaching "bonk." She also enjoys things like Twizzlers and Neccos for a quick burst of pure sugar. Maybe not the best nutrition, according to Blessing, but she is a true believer in taking along food that she wants to eat; otherwise food can be hard to force down when your mouth is dry from breathing hard.

Ultrarunner Jim Garcia's trademark food is a mixture of mashed potatoes, baked beans, and Texas Pete (a Louisiana hot sauce). He occasionally eats homemade Korean rice balls (the equivalent of a California sushi roll) that he carries with him in a baggie placed in a pouch or in his shorts' pocket. The night before his 14:35:27 Rocky Raccoon 100-mile performance, he put some Boston Market mashed potatoes and gravy in a camping squeeze tube and kept it on ice in his drop bag. The tube was easy to grab from the bag and eat on the fly.

Tom Sobal considers the plants and fruits growing along the trail on his runs to be wild aid stations. He recalls foraging bananas and guavas on a trail run in Hawaii, eating apricots and service berries in Utah, apples in the Midwest, and cherries in Europe. An advantage of trail running is that these fruits are usually okay to eat if they are located on public lands.

When Cynci Calvin was new to trail racing, she found herself lingering at various race aid stations positively overwhelmed by the buffet selection. She particularly enjoyed the little boiled and salted new potatoes served cold along with cold tortellini pasta. A few potatoes and pasta combined with a couple of nice fizzy swigs of Coca-Cola had her "hittin' the next segment of the trail like a mountain goat being chased by a cougar.

"Everyone is so different. Just because Coke and potatoes work for me doesn't mean it will work for someone else. At the Western States Endurance Run (sometimes called a 100-mile-long buffet), I've seen everything from folks perfectly content with gels and liquid protein supplements like Ensure to those who demand that their crew deliver them a cheeseburger and milkshake at the 60-mile point. These folks have learned what works for them by experimenting, and have more enjoyable runs as the result."

Cramping is a problem for many athletes. Experimentation results in various remedies. One of the few things Kristin Jossi can tolerate throughout challenging races such as Alaska's Crow Pass Crossing and Resurrection Pass 50 Miler is potato cubes. Since sweets often make her nauseous, she eats undercooked cubes (they stay a bit crunchy and don't fall apart) with a little salt and pepper. They stuff easily into a Ziploc bag in a waist pack, are easy to pinch out with uncoordinated fingers, are easy to chew, go well with water or Gatorade, and their consistency is not influenced by temperature changes. Jossi also carries lighter-weight foods like raisins, miniature Snickers, and salted pretzel sticks.

Mark Nesfeder eats fig bars and cinnamon raisin bagels on his longer forays, whether training or racing. He finds fig bars very light yet filling, and not too heavy in his stomach—they never give him digestive problems. He was hoping to snack on similar treats during the first Mount Elbert Snowshoe Challenge in 1994, but he found everything at the aid station had frozen solid in the subzero temperatures. He warmed up his frozen fig bars and bagel chunks by stuffing them between his jacket and Capilene underwear. As for his frozen water bottle, a few whacks and he dislodged the ice buildup with some success.

For his longer runs David Wise likes to put a Starburst or fruit-flavored Tootsie Roll between his cheek and gum to keep his mouth from getting dry . . . and to add a little sugar.

Brandy Erholtz, USATF Mountain Runner of the Year 2008, says she has a hard time eating on the run. "Luckily this isn't a problem until I start

Here are some thoughts on nutrition and training from Kami Semick, USATF Trail Champion (at various distances):

My mantra is to eat as close to the earth as possible. I've heard this referred to as a "whole foods"–based diet. What this translates to is focusing my calories on minimally handled and processed foods. Anything that is not in a wrapper is fair game, be it meat, fruits, vegetables, grains, or fats. I also don't cut out categories of food. If animal flesh looks appealing, I eat it. Certain dairy items are a big part of my diet. And I consume a large amount of nut- and vegetable-based fats.

One of my biggest shifts in thinking regarding food, which has led me to be able to recover faster, avoid injury, and train harder, was an increase in protein intake. The amino acids found in high-quality protein are the building blocks needed to repair damaged muscles. I make sure I have protein from a quality source at each meal, and my snacks contain a protein element. Whole eggs and egg whites are typically in my breakfast, whole milk plain yogurts, cottage cheese, or leftover meats from dinner are a highlight for lunch, and quality fish or chicken are what I focus on for dinner. Granted I'm not a very exciting chef. But whole grains, leafy greens, vegetables, and protein always make it on my plate.

There has also been a focus lately on leafy greens. My husband is a talented organic gardener and supplies our family with a variety of leafy greens six out of twelve months of the year.

On supplements: All of USADA's (U.S. Anti-Doping Agency) literature will warn athletes away from supplements. But speaking for myself, it is close to impossible to take in all of the minerals and vitamins my body needs in order to handle the demands of ultrarunning. Even with a whole foods–based diet, I find myself needing supplements for iron, calcium, and Vitamin D. I think the key with supplements is buying from a quality source. Sometimes that means talking to a sport nutritionist who can guide you toward high-quality sources.

doing ultras." When Erholtz makes that transition, she could learn something from Blake Norwood, race director of North Carolina's Umstead 100 Miler, who has written an article on how to train for and run your first ultra. "The long run must incorporate eating and drinking training and experimentation. More runners are lost due to lack of energy from not eating properly than from muscle fatigue. You need to train your body to process food and liquid while on the run and train how to eat, if not on the run, then at least on the walk. I believe it is difficult to run 100 miles on just gel packs and energy drinks. Most folks get so tired of just one or two items that the mere mention of them later in the race makes them sick. Become familiar with a wide variety of foods. Later in the race, foods that are easy to swallow become more important. I find that canned peaches and pears, milk, and ice cream work well for me; find out what works well for you and never pass a staffed aid station without eating and drinking."

Anita Ortiz, 2009 winner of the Western States 100 Miler and Pikes Peak Marathon, has made the transition from shorter distance events— she has been a top-ten finisher in the World Mountain Trophy Race at the 8-kilometer distance. Lately she has started running ultras and has had to change her food intake accordingly. "I never used to eat, or hydrate on my runs. Of course I never ran for more than 15 miles at one time. Now I'm running longer distances and I know I need to hydrate and take in calories. It took a lot of experimentation to figure out what worked for me. Once I tried peanut butter but I couldn't keep it down. Then I tried bagels and that didn't work either. It felt like I had a rock in my stomach. PowerGels, watermelon, and Coke seem to work best for me. During Western I ate thirty-eight PowerGels and my gut felt great."

CHAPTER 9

Injuries and Injury Prevention

Injuries are something everyone strives to avoid . . . often to such a degree that they shun thinking, or even saying, the word *injury* or, alternatively, reach the point of obsessing over them. Fortunately, trail runners tend to be a relatively healthy lot, and running on soft surfaces reduces the likelihood of certain types of injury. Then again, sometimes trail running is indeed a contact sport. Unlike the typical and seemingly mundane repetitive stress injuries suffered by road runners, trail runners are known to adorn themselves with surface lacerations that are much more fascinating than tendonitis, shin splints, or chondromalacia, which are not visible to the naked eye. Yet, a mishap with the trail, a tree, rocks, a cliff, or some ice is just as likely to result in a subtle overuse problem as it is in a more dramatic flesh wound. Trail runners are not invincible. They do, from time to time, suffer injuries and even fall prey to the same overuse problems that plague road runners.

ACUTE INJURIES

Serious traumas, strains, tears, or ruptures are types of acute injuries that cause bleeding, swelling, discoloration, or impair muscle function and performance. Even worse, acute injuries can result in broken bones, infection, loss of consciousness, blindness, and other maladies. The consequences of suffering such an acute trail running injury are only made more severe by the fact that most trails are in remote, hard-to-reach areas where it is difficult to either evacuate an injured runner or bring emergency care to the site of the injury.

Severe acute injuries are likely to require medical attention. In contrast, common trail running trauma—strained joints from sudden efforts to avoid falling, and abrasions and bruising from falls that were not avoided—are usually remedied by rest and ice. When possible, end a trail run near a cool body of water, such as a stream, river, or mountain pond, that can be used for an invigorating and therapeutic soak. Elevating one's legs after a hard effort also helps to flush the blood from the battered muscle tissue and reduce inflammation. Compression socks, calf sleeves, or tights also help with pushing blood out of your recovering lower leg muscles.

Twisted (or Rolled) Ankles

Twisted or rolled ankles are dreaded by all trail runners. A momentary lapse of concentration, a misstep, a shaded divot, some slippery mud or ice, or simple lack of coordination is all that it takes to cause an ankle to twist or roll. Depending on the severity, a twisted or rolled ankle can result in minor muscle tears, swelling, tendon and ligament damage, or even broken bones. If the twist or roll results in substantial pain and swelling, it is a good idea to consult with a medical professional to determine the seriousness of the injury.

The best treatment for ankle problems is to avoid them by strengthening the muscles that support the ankle and working on flexibility of the area through stretching. If you are vulnerable to ankle twists or rolls, then wear trail shoes with higher ankle collars, or wrap or tape your ankles for additional support. Consult with a trainer, physical therapist, or other health care professional to learn proper ankle taping techniques.

Torn Ligaments

Ligaments work to join bones together. Certain knee ligaments, known by their three-letter abbreviations, have become infamous because of a few other three-letter abbreviations including NFL, NBA, NHL, etc. The ACL (anterior cruciate ligament) and the PCL (posterior cruciate ligament) are found within the knee joint and prevent the femur from sliding too much on the tibia. Trail runners are most prone to a rupture of the ACL when a foot planted on uneven ground forces the leg to rotate excessively at the knee.

Jay Hodde, MS, ATC, and a columnist for *UltraRunning* magazine, points out that trail runners who run on rutted, rocky, and root-infested trails stand an increased likelihood of suffering a twisting injury to the knee. In addition to ACL ruptures, Hodde warns that a sharp, deep pain within the knee joint may be a tear to the meniscus, which can be debilitating. The meniscii absorb the shock transferred to the tibia from the femur and help distribute body weight throughout the knee. A tear to the meniscus results from a distinct, traumatic event, such as a mis-step that causes a twist to the knee while it is in a slightly bent position, when the shearing forces are at their highest level.

A torn meniscus causes instability, swelling, pain, and the inability to run due to a "catching" or "locking" sensation in the knee upon attempting to bend or straighten the joint. The standard treatment of ice, rest, compression, elevation, and anti-inflammatories is recommended as the first line of defense in treating a torn meniscus. Hodde advises seeing a trained physician to determine the extent of the tear, because continuing to run on a small tear may increase the size of the tear and ultimately damage the meniscus enough that it becomes irreparable. Certainly, take time off from running and look to alternative activities that do not require repetitive knee flexion and extension. For rehabilitation, use pain as an indicator of when a cross-training exercise aggravates the tear. Stretching and strengthening the quadriceps and hamstrings will help to keep the damage to a minimum.

Other Acute Injuries

In addition to the foregoing more common acute trail running injuries, trail runners should be aware of the risk of poking an eye, breaking a bone, being lacerated or punctured, or otherwise being harmed in a mishap on the trails. Although the medical response and emergency handling of such calamities is beyond the scope of this book, it is strongly advised that you read up or receive training on wilderness first aid and in-the-field medical care and CPR before venturing out to run the trails.

OVERUSE INJURIES

Overuse injuries are caused by various factors, including incorrect running form, running on shoes that have lost their cushioning and support, or long, jarring descents on rocky, compacted, or other hard surfaces, especially when the leg muscles are already fatigued so that they do not absorb the impact as readily.

Muscle strains are a type of overuse injury caused by overstretching muscle fiber and can range from minor microtears to more severe tears or ruptures in deeper muscle tissue. Minor strains manifest themselves through pain and post-trauma stiffness. Depending on the severity of a strain, treatment can be anything from pre-run warm-up and stretching and post-run ice applications to massage to medical treatment and rehabilitation.

Blisters

Blisters are, perhaps, the quintessential trail running overuse injury. Blisters develop when friction causes two layers of skin to rub against each other to the point where the outer epidermis layer separates from the deeper layers. The sac between the layers usually fills with lymph fluid, although it may fill with blood when the blister is deep or increasingly stressed. Blisters are caused by any combination of friction, heat, and moisture.

The best way to treat blisters is to try to prevent them in the first place. Blister prevention may involve any one or a combination of the following: foot powder to keep your feet dry, lubrication (petroleum jelly, Bag Balm, or special sports lubricants sold at specialty running shoe stores) between your toes and on the ball of the foot, wool or other moisture-wicking socks, thin socks, double layer socks, changing into dry socks, shoe changes within a run or race, buying shoes that fit or shoes that allow for foot swelling, trimmed toenails, orthotics, foot pads, foot taping, altered shoe lacing, insoles, running gaiters, proper hydration to reduce foot swelling, and taking the time to clear gravel, sand, and other debris from your shoes.

Inevitably, blisters will occur, so it is important to know how to treat them. Smaller blisters do not necessarily need any treatment other than lubrication and a bandage. It is often the case that the fluid will be reabsorbed. Generally, for larger blisters that are more than ¾ inch in size, draining them will be more comfortable, assuming they are clear or white. The proper treatment involves wiping the blistered area with an alcohol pad and, at a point closest to the skin, lancing the blister with a flame-sterilized needle. Drain the fluid, clean the entire area, leaving the outer skin intact to cover the soft skin beneath, and cover it with a bandage.

Do not lance blood blisters. Lancing a blood blister could cause infection through direct contact with the blood. Simply clean and then lubricate the surface of the blood blister and cover it with a bandage. You may choose from a variety of bandages and moleskin-type products that are now available on the market. Depending on particular use, types of blisters, skin conditions, climate, etc., different products will be more successful than others, so try a variety.

Black Toenails

Like blisters, black toenails are a common trail running affliction. Toenails turn black as the result of bleeding under the nail, caused by pressure from—usually on descents—or impact with the shoe's toe box. Black toenails may result from shoes that are either too large, so the foot slides and smashes into the front of the shoe on descents, or too small, so the toes are crushed by pressure from the toe box. As the blood under the nail dries it turns dark, and depending on the extent of the pressure and impact to the toenail, the nail may "die" and eventually fall off when a new toenail grows underneath and pushes it out, much the way a baby tooth is replaced by adult teeth. According to Bill Hilty, MD, a trail runner who practices emergency medicine in Grand Junction, Colorado, the decision of whether to run after suffering black toenails should be driven by the amount of pain that running causes. "Use your pain gauge to determine whether the damage is severe enough that running and the associated trauma would cause further damage."

Chafing

Although chafing is more of an overuse "annoyance" than an injury, try telling that to someone who suffers a bad enough rash that they cannot run for days until the chafed area heals. Usually suffered in the inner thigh and armpit area, chafing is merely a skin abrasion caused by the friction and heat of skin rubbing against skin or clothing. To prevent chafing, wear clothes that do not have seams in areas prone to abrasion and apply skin lubrication before running. In addition to petroleum jelly and Bag Balm, there are a handful of new skin lubes available on the market designed specifically for runners.

Tendonitis

Tendonitis, the inflammation of tendons, is another injury caused by overuse and improper running form. Tendons, which attach muscle to bone, can become sore and flare up to the point where they no longer glide back and forth in their protective sheaths, resulting in pain and possible seizure. Common areas for trail runners to suffer tendonitis are in the ankle, the knee, and the Achilles tendon, which is the large tendon that attaches the calf muscles to the heel bone. Achilles tendonitis is caused by overworking the calf muscle to the point where it becomes weak and shifts too much of the body weight to the Achilles tendon. Achilles tendonitis may result from a dramatic increase in hill running or an abrupt switch from road running to trail running. Another type of tendonitis, hamstring tendonitis, is often the result of overstriding, hill running, or inflexibility of the hamstring.

As with many overuse injuries, tendonitis can be chronic yet ignored or "run through," because the pain often subsides once the affected area is warmed through exercise. Tendonitis is, however, likely to get more painful as the run progresses, and after the run it often results in soreness, pain, weakness, and stiffness. Achilles tendonitis may show up in the form of swelling, sensitivity to the ankle area, and possibly a grating sensation in the heel. As an overuse injury, the cure is to lay off running for a while, although pre-run warm-up and stretching and post-run ice and massage may help, depending on the severity of the injury. Shoes that have ample forefoot flex, heel lifts, orthotics, and calf strengthening exercises may help to decrease the load that is borne by the Achilles tendon. Hamstring tendonitis may be avoided through an effective stretching and strengthening routine that focuses on the hamstring muscles.

Stress Fractures

Stress fractures are less likely to haunt trail runners than they are road runners because they are commonly caused by overuse through repetitive shock on unforgiving surfaces—read "roads." Runners with eating disorders and particularly women with calcium deficiencies are predisposed to stress fractures, which are hairline breaks in a foot, ankle, shin, thigh, or even pelvic bone. Stress fractures often manifest themselves as a sensitive spot that is painful to the touch. They are likely to begin as dull aches and, if not detected and addressed, develop into sharp, persistent pain that becomes more severe during a run.

Like most overuse injuries, the proper treatment for stress fractures is to rest the tender area and relieve the pressure, which in most cases means taking time off from running. Depending on the nature of the stress fracture, the "rest" period may allow for non-weight-bearing cross training with such activities as swimming, aqua jogging, bicycling, rowing, rock climbing, and other athletic pursuits that do not expose the affected area to pressure. More severe stress fractures require a month or two of immobilization through the use of a walking cast or "boot."

Following a realistic training program that allows for a gradual increase in distance and intensity can help your body adapt better to the increasing demands placed on it. Alternating your running surfaces and seeking out softer surfaces such as trails can reduce impact stress on the foot, as can wearing appropriate running shoes for your foot type and replacing them before they are significantly worn out.
—Perry H. Julien, DPM, "The Painful Heel" in *Marathon & Beyond*

Plantar Fasciitis

Often mis-self-diagnosed by trail runners as a bone bruise, plantar fasciitis is an inflammation of the fascia—the dense band of connective tissue that attaches the bottom of the heel to the metatarsal heads or ball of the foot and helps to give the foot its arched shape, stability, alignment, shock absorption, propulsion, and resilience. Plantar fasciitis is often caused by poor arch support and can be remedied by stretching the Achilles tendon and strengthening calf and foot muscles to provide better arch strength. Less proactive remedies include wearing orthotics or arch supports, or taping the foot to take stress off the fascia. Icing the foot after running also helps with recovery.

Shin Splints

Shin splints—the misnomer for what is more properly classified as posterior tibial tendonitis or strain—is an injury that is more likely to plague
road runners, especially flat-footed ones, than trail runners. Shin splints
cause pain that runs along the front of the shin. The pain emanates from
the muscle that runs along the inner edge of the shinbone and attaches
to tendons at the bottom of the foot, behind the anklebone. If the foot
flattens too much, it causes tremendous stress on the tendons and trans-
mits pain to the shin area, even though that is not actually the place
where the damage occurs. Runners who attempt to increase their mileage too quickly, who run in worn-out shoes, who overpronate, or who
run with more weight than normal are more susceptible to shin splints.
Pre-run heat and post-run ice on the entire lower leg and fresh shoes
may help for minor shin splints, although strengthening the muscles
that support the foot and building up arch strength or wearing arch supports or orthotics may be necessary.

General Knee Pain

Although trails and their forgiving, soft surfaces and diverse footing are
much better for the whole body than are roads, hilly trails take a toll
on the knees, especially when we storm the descents with bad form.
There are a number of knee injuries that tend to pester trail runners.
One, known as chondromalacia, "runner's knee," or "patello-femoral
syndrome," is the grating pain under the patella or kneecap. It is caused
when the patella is pulled out of alignment with the groove at the bottom of the thighbone. The effect of chondromalacia is that the cartilage
under the patella softens and causes soreness and swelling in the area.
The injury can result from torque of the shinbone that is sometimes due
to foot misalignment, weak arches, an imbalance between quadriceps
and hamstring strength, wide hips, or severe overpronation. Mild cases
of chondromalacia may be remedied by rest, ice, and strengthening the
quadriceps, while more acute cases require more invasive solutions from
a sports medicine professional.

Knee tendons are also an area prone to trail running injuries. The iliotibial band ("IT band") is a thick band of connective tissue on the outside

or lateral side of the leg that runs from the upper gluteal muscles and outer thigh down to the side of the knee to above the shin. IT band syndrome occurs when repetitive friction from the band's sliding over the lateral end of the femur causes it to become inflamed. Pain is felt on the outside of the knee and usually increases (sometimes to the point of debilitation) about ten minutes into a run. It is a relatively common injury, suffered by more than 10 percent of all runners, and is often brought on by long descents on hard surfaces. When caught at an early stage the syndrome can be remedied without too much downtime. However, if not detected or blatantly ignored, IT band syndrome will sideline the trail runner. IT band syndrome can be prevented through the use of running shoes that are appropriate for a trail runner's particular needs and particular running form. Special stretches, mentioned in Chapter 6, also help to hold the syndrome at bay.

Be alert to the symptoms of an injury. Know the difference between discomfort and pain. Pain is often the body's way of putting the mind on notice in an effort to prevent further and lasting damage. Learn to constantly monitor body parts and distinguish between discomfort ("good pain"), which is the result of sore muscles rebuilding themselves, and injury-related pain ("bad pain"), which should not be ignored. Generally, sharp, persistent pain that shows up and remains in a specific area of the body is not something that can be run through or neglected. Such pain is likely a sign that something is seriously out of whack, and a runner who experiences such abnormalities should stop running and consult with a health care practitioner.

AVOIDING AND RECOVERING FROM INJURIES

One of the first rules in dealing with trail running injuries is to avoid them by learning to detect injury at the earliest onset, at which point it becomes necessary to adjust running form, training, and/or racing schedule. Depending on the type of injury, it may even be necessary to lay off running to prevent a niggling pain from developing into a full-blown injury. Unfortunately, sensing an injury before it gets painful, swollen, or worse requires highly developed physiological insight—one that often only comes at the expense of learning from the school of hard knocks.

The best, most complete recovery from a specific trail running injury is a full and permanent one. Remembering what caused the injury and keeping a logbook or some sort of documentation of the injury and recuperation processes will be a great resource in the event the problem returns in the future. By being able to look at a record of what relieved pain, whether or not the injury was exacerbated by running, and how the body responded to different remedies, you'll have the best possible tool for nipping the problem in the bud, should it flare up.

Rest

Although different injuries require different treatment, there are a handful of universal remedies and preventive measures that apply to the injuries discussed above. Resting, the first best cure, is probably the hardest prescription for runners to swallow. There's the old joke about the patient who visits a doctor saying, "Doc, it hurts when I do this" and the doctor replies, "So, don't do that." As obvious as it may be to nonrunners, runners struggle with the concept that the best thing to do when a running-related injury flares up is to decrease or stop running.

A day or two off from running does not necessarily mean a day or two off from all exercise. While it may be enough to prevent a running injury from becoming a major setback, time away from running does not have to cut into a runner's fitness base. Depending on the nature of the injury, the "rest" can be an active rest that may include resistance training and cross-training activities that do not exacerbate the injury or delay recovery. Resting may even allow for some running, albeit less or with less intensity, so long as it does not cause pain, inflammation, overcompensation of another body part, or otherwise increase soreness or retard recovery. The trick is to start resting as early as possible, usually at the first sign of soreness. Certainly rest is the best cure when the injury is from a traumatic event, such as a sprain or twist. Heeding early warning signs requires sensitivity gained through experience, a level of discipline, and an understanding of the benefits that the time off will provide in the big picture. The length of the rest period depends on the severity and type of injury but should be at least long enough for the pain to subside.

Ice

Another somewhat universal injury treatment is to promote healing and recovery with ice or cold water. Ice and cold water serve as natural anti-inflammatories by causing blood to leave the exposed area, thereby reducing swelling. The reduced swelling will numb and decrease pain and may have the benefit of reducing the impact of an injury.

It is best to cool or ice an injury as soon as possible after suffering the injury or after completing a workout or race. As an effective injury prevention or recovery technique, many trail runners sit, wade, or swim in cool ponds, lakes, rivers, stream pools, or other bodies of water after a run. Depending on water temperature, depth, flow, and one's threshold for dealing with cold, a therapeutic soak may entail several short intervals or a ten- to fifteen-minute sit. Unlike water, ice can be applied directly to the affected area (or above the injury, if a bandage, cast, or other barrier prevents access). Use an ice bag, a bag of frozen vegetables (peas and corn work very well), or chemical cold packs. To avoid frostbite, do not place the ice directly on the skin. Ice until the area is generally numb, but not longer than twenty minutes at a time. Sometimes it is recommended to ice an injury before a run, but consult a sports medicine professional to determine whether to run when injured.

Pain Relief and Anti-inflammatory Medicines

The decision of whether to use aspirin, ibuprofen, or other nonsteroidal anti-inflammatory drugs is a personal one. While runners can and do abuse such drugs as a means of deadening pain to get them through a training session or race, anti-inflammatories are nonetheless seen by many as effective aids for limiting swelling and pain. You should be aware of the potential risks that are associated with anti-inflammatories, especially when the drugs are taken in great quantities, on an empty stomach, or when you are dehydrated. Rhabdomyolysis is a breakdown of skeletal muscle caused when myoglobin, a protein stored in muscle fibers, is released into the blood and flows into the kidneys, causing them to fail. Studies have shown that the chances of suffering rhabdomyolysis are increased by the use of anti-inflammatories, especially when running in hot weather when dehydrated.

Homeopathic and Other Remedies

Arnica montana, a homeopathic remedy that is taken either orally or topically, is used to counter the effects of bruises, traumas, muscle fatigue, and pain. Arnica has been proven in double-blind studies to help smooth out the rough edges that are often caused by strenuous exercise—swelling, muscle fatigue, and stiffness. Other remedial or therapeutic measures for sore muscles and fatigued or strained soft tissue include heat rubs, hot tubs, saunas, steam rooms, and similar spa-like treatments. Generally, heat should not be used as a treatment until internal bleeding has dissipated, which is typically three days after an injury occurs. Acupuncture, rolfing or structural integration, applied kinesiology, chiropractic treatment, naturopathic, homeopathic, or herbal remedies, acupressure, and many other non-Western healing arts offer trail runners a wide variety of alternatives when it comes to finding a remedy for or preventing an injury.

Sports massage is a common therapy for runners, whether it is used to prevent injury, treat injury, or merely to enhance or maintain performance. Massage therapy can have any one of or a combination of benefits. It can improve circulation and aid the body's muscles to cleanse themselves of built-up toxins. Massage can relieve pressure points in muscle tissue caused by a blocked blood flow or poor posture by helping to adjust body alignment. It can reduce muscle spasms by assisting muscle tissue to be soft, supple, and elongated. Choose a massage therapist that has been properly trained and certified, especially in sports massage, and if at all possible, go to a therapist who comes with strong referrals from trail runners and, if possible, also is a trail runner.

Common-Sense Cure

Trail runners who suffer certain types of overuse/soft-tissue injuries are often surprised by the almost miraculous recovery they experience by adopting and incorporating a regular stretching, resistance training, and cross-training regimen into their training. Many of the injuries discussed in the first part of this chapter are caused by tight soft and connective tissue, muscle imbalances and weaknesses, and simple overuse of body parts that are traumatized by running. Similarly, improving running form and general base fitness, strength, and flexibility combine to serve as the best lines of defense against running injuries. Taking a holistic approach, injury prevention includes eating a proper diet, getting enough sleep, and maintaining a healthy lifestyle. A runner who is overstressed from work may run with tight muscles and rigid posture and will be more susceptible to injury than a relaxed runner.

Although a trail running injury is likely to be accompanied—if not defined—by physical pain, often the greatest suffering from an injury is that it translates into time away from trail running. Do not underestimate the psychological and emotional aspects of an injury, because it is often the "need" to run for psychological and emotional reasons that drives trail runners to run themselves into injury in the first place. With the onset of an injury, it is easy to lose perspective and feel as though any time away from running will be devastating to one's fitness. As a result, ignoring or "training through" the injury is sometimes seen as a more attractive option than pursuing some cross-training activity that allows for recuperation and recovery.

In an article on the subject of the psychological and emotional aspects of running injuries, *UltraRunning* columnists Kevin Setnes and Kris Clark Setnes observe that when "an injury occurs, causing an abrupt cessation of the positive benefits, athletes may experience post-injury psychological and emotional disturbance. Some sports psychologists have suggested injured athletes progress through a grief cycle similar to that which is experienced by the terminally ill." The article cites a study in which a group of "prevented runners" who were unable to run for two weeks due to injury showed signs of depression, anxiety, confusion, and low self-esteem. The loss of running deprived the subjects of coping mechanisms and stress-management strategies, leaving them tense, disturbed, moody, angry, and lethargic.

Granted, running trails may well be one of life's better experiences, but it is important to maintain a sense of perspective and realize that although Ben Franklin was a bit plump to run trails, his maxim that "a stitch in time saves nine" applies directly to many types of overuse and stress injuries. A day or two of mountain biking, Nordic skiing, swimming, rock climbing, or some other pursuit that involves endurance and the outdoors is not all that bad, especially when it expedites the return to healthier trail running. Take the time to improve life outside of running. Spend it with family and friends. Volunteer to help build or maintain a local trail. Read a good book, practice yoga, see a movie, write some letters, weed the garden, or clean or fix things that need it.

To be a holistic injury-free trail runner, learn how to read your body's first warnings and show the good sense of listening to those signs and easing up, or take time off from running to allow for necessary rest. Maintain a big-picture outlook and realize that nipping an injury in the bud requires a bit of psychological and emotional fortitude that ends up paying big dividends in the long run, so to speak. Being a healthy trail runner not only requires laying off trail running at the first onset of injury, but also demands the discipline of resisting the urge to return to the trails before full recovery.

Unfortunately, it is hard to know exactly when it is safe to return to running without causing re-injury. Do not test the waters by taking anti-inflammatories or icing before a run. That will only numb or mask the injury in the event that the return to running was premature. It takes understanding your body, and that understanding is often gained by experience through trial and error. There is also the challenge of knowing how hard to come back, especially if the time away from running was substantial. This will depend on the type of injury and how severe it was, as well as the fitness level going into and maintained during the injury. Keep the return to training in perspective, and try not to go back too quickly at the risk of re-injury. While a base of experience and fitness makes for a solid foundation for training, trail running abilities are neither lost nor regained overnight.

CHAPTER 10

Hazards of the Trail

Since you can encounter any number of elements, surprises, and hazards on the trail, it's important to be prepared. If you're on a long run in the mountains, expect variable weather conditions. If the run is in a remote area, expect to see animals—some friendly, some not so friendly. Depending on the season, plants can grow out of control, encroach on the trail, and when in contact with human skin, can cause minor or major skin irritations. If the trail is easily accessible, there's always the possibility of running into someone who could be there for reasons other than enjoying its use. Without a map, getting lost can lead to panic or physical dangers that could include dehydration, hypothermia, or altitude sickness. Although some dangers are inherent in the sport, planning ahead and being cautious and aware of your surroundings at all times greatly enhance the trail running experience.

WEATHER

Consider this familiar Colorado saying: "If you don't like the weather, wait five minutes and it will change." Not a very comforting thought for a runner in the midst of a trail run who didn't think to prepare for potential weather changes. Less comforting is the fact that storms approach as quickly on the Appalachian Trail or in the plains of Kansas as they do in the Colorado Rockies. The best advice for trail runners is to be prepared for any condition, especially if the run is a long one in a remote area.

Hypothermia

Weather hazards vary, depending on the season and the region. If you are exposed to severe cold without enough protection, then you are a prime candidate for hypothermia, a condition that occurs when body temperature drops below 95°F. The onset of symptoms is usually slow, with a gradual loss of mental acuity and physical ability. Additional symptoms include drowsiness, loss of coordination, uncontrollable shivering, and pale and cold skin. The person experiencing hypothermia, in fact, may be unaware that he or she is in a state that requires emergency medical treatment. Another unpleasant condition that arises from extreme cold is frostbite, which causes tissue damage primarily to extremities and exposed flesh.

Frostbite

There are three stages of frostbite including frostnip, superficial frost-bite, and deep frostbite. Frostnip looks pale, feels cold, and is similar in physiology to a first-degree burn. Passive skin-to-skin contact is the best out-in-the-field warming method for frostnip. Superficial frostbite causes the skin to feel numb, waxy, and frozen as ice crystals form in the skin cells while the rest of the skin remains flexible. Superficial frostbite may result in blisters within twenty-four hours after rewarming. Treatment for second-degree or superficial frostbite is rapid rewarming by immersion in warm (104° to 108°F) water. Unlike frostnip, the injury should not be rewarmed by simple application of heat. Proper rewarming is crucial to healing. Since frostnip and superficial frostbite can look almost identical prior to rewarming, it is not recommended that any heat be applied to any suspected frostbite other than skin to skin or the warm-water treat-ment described above.

Deep frostbite is the most serious stage of frostbite. In this stage, blood vessels, muscles, tendons, nerves, and bone may be frozen. This stage will lead to permanent damage, blood clots, and sometimes, in severe cases, gangrene. No feeling is experienced in the affected area, the skin feels hard, and there is usually no blistering after rewarming. Loss of tissue to some extent is guaranteed in deep frostbite. However, even with deep frostbite, some frozen limbs may be saved if medical attention is obtained as soon as possible. In all stages avoid massaging the affected area and avoid application of high radiant heat sources such as the heat from stoves and fires.

Wet clothes, high winds and the resulting wind chill, poor circula-tion, fatigue, and poor fluid and food intake exacerbate frostbite. In cold temperatures, wear suitable clothing with appropriate layering and protect more exposed areas such as hands, feet, ears, and head. (See Chapter 7 for specific gear suggestions.)

Sunburn

If you are unprepared during warmer months, then the combination of heat, humidity, and sun can be harmful to you. Sunburn, heat cramps, heat exhaustion, and heatstroke are all potential hazards. Sunburn and heat cramps can be self-treated in most cases, but heat exhaustion and heatstroke are much more serious and may render a victim helpless.

Sunburn from prolonged exposure can go from mild to severe, resulting in blisters, fever, and headaches. One should be prepared to use sunblock and to reapply the product as long as exposure continues in order to avoid these discomforts. To treat sunburn, take a shower using soap to remove oils that may block pores and prevent the body from cooling naturally. If blisters occur, apply dry, sterile dressings and seek medical attention. Sunscreen with a high SPF number is an essential addition to every trail runner's fanny pack. One that is billed as a "performance" sunscreen is best since the breathability is important to an athlete.

Heat Cramps, Heat Exhaustion, and Heatstroke

The symptoms of heat cramps are painful spasms usually in leg and abdominal muscles, often coupled with heavy sweating. To relieve a spasm, apply firm pressure or gently massage the cramping muscles. Sip water unless drinking causes nausea, in which case cease drinking.

Symptoms of heat exhaustion include heavy sweating, weakness, cold, pale, and clammy skin, fainting, and weakened pulse, even though it is possible to have a normal temperature. A heat exhaustion victim should be taken to a cool place to lie down, clothing should be loosened, and cool, wet cloths should be applied. Placing ice cubes or plastic bags filled with cold water in the armpits and the crotch also proves beneficial in bringing down the victim's temperature. Be careful, however, to make sure the ice is removed from time to time to prevent frostbite (especially in the crotch). If vomiting occurs, seek immediate medical attention.

Heatstroke is a severe medical emergency that is indicated by high body temperature (over 106°F) and further identified by hot dry skin, a rapid strong pulse, possible loss of consciousness, and absence of or very little sweating. Immediately move a heatstroke victim to a cooler environment and try a cool bath, sponging, or the ice treatment described above to decrease the body temperature, but *do not give fluids.* Delaying a trip to the hospital can be fatal.

Dehydration

No matter what the weather, dehydration is always a potential hazard. As related earlier in the nutrition section, drink early and often, and be sure the liquid is pure. Don't stop on a trail run to drink unfiltered water from a lake or stream, even if the water appears to run clear—clear running water is no indication that the water is free from contaminants. Giardiasis (a condition caused by drinking water contaminated by feces) may not show up in the human system for days or even weeks after ingestion of contaminated water, and the effects are rather unpleasant, including gas, bloating, loss of appetite, diarrhea, and cramps. Boiling will rid the water of most pathogens but is usually not a convenient method. Carrying a water filter or iodine tablets makes more sense for the trail runner.

Lightning

Although extreme temperatures can prove bothersome and even life threatening on the trail, inclement weather, including lightning and thunderstorms, can be an equal menace. According to the National Lightning Safety Institute (NLSI) based in Louisville, Colorado, lightning causes more deaths in the United States than any other natural hazard. Florida ranks as the top state for lightning-related injuries and death. The National Oceanic and Atmospheric Administration published lightning statistics in the United States gathered between 1959 and 1994, ranking July as having the most lightning incidents, followed by June and August, respectively.

Regardless of the month or region, no place is absolutely safe from lightning. The NLSI offers the following personal lightning safety tips: Lightning often precedes rain, so don't wait for the rain to begin before you stop running; where possible, find shelter in a substantial building or in a car, truck, or a van with the windows completely shut; avoid open spaces, water, and high ground; avoid metal objects including electric wires, fences, machinery, motors, power tools, etc. Beneath canopies, small picnic or rain shelters, and near trees are also unsafe places to be when there's lightning. If lightning is striking nearby, crouch down with feet together and hands placed over ears to minimize any hearing damage from thunder. The threat of lightning is often perceived by the senses when body hair feels as if it is standing on end. In this case immediately drop to the ground and lie flat. Avoid being closer than 15 feet to other people, and avoid running for thirty minutes after the last perceived lightning or thunder. When thunderstorms are in the area, but not directly overhead, the lightning threat can exist even when it is sunny or when clear sky is visible.

FLORA AND FAUNA

Trail runners often venture into areas teeming with wildlife. The potential for animal sightings varies with the season, region, terrain, as well as the amount of human traffic on a particular route. Even if a run is void of an animal encounter, scat, broken tree limbs, or carcasses can provide remnant evidence of animal presence along a trail. Consider this warning from Kevin Sanders, wildlife biologist and Yellowstone naturalist: "When you leave the road and are in a true wilderness area, you become a member of the food chain."

Sanders says the unpredictability of bears, bison, and mountain lions pose the most danger to the trail runner, especially a trail runner that is unprepared for potential animal encounters. Be aware of the wildlife populations in any area in which you plan to run. Take the time to gather information and educate yourself on the best way to react during an encounter.

Bears

Fatal encounters with bears are exacerbated by a common mistake people make—staring at the ground while walking or running and being unaware of the surroundings. This is certainly true for the trail runner who runs with eyes cast downward, hoping to avoid a misstep along the route. The majority of people don't notice a bear until they are within

14 feet, much too close for comfort and leaving little time to evaluate the situation and respond in a thoughtful, appropriate manner. So try to stay alert. The strategy in a black bear encounter is to stop immediately, stand still, pick up a stick or rock, and prepare to fight. Aggressive behavior is the best approach. However, the opposite is true if the bear is a grizzly. Act calmly in a grizzly encounter. If the bear is close and acts aggressively, stand still. Don't make eye contact, talk softly, walk very slowly backward, toss a hat or coat on the ground toward the bear to diffuse its interest, and as a last resort lie down, curl up in the fetal position, covering your neck with your hands, and play dead.

The only state void of bears is Hawaii, and since the species are not true hibernators, sightings are not seasonal, although the chance of an encounter is greater in the spring and summer. Females or sows will attack to protect their cubs and are typically less tolerant of human presence than males are.

Preventative measures for the single runner to avert potential conflicts with bears include clapping, talking loudly, or chanting. The jury is still out on wearing bells, which have been known to attract curious bears. A proven deterrent is bear spray consisting of cayenne pepper. However, a downside exists to spraying in inclement weather because rain, wind, and snow may reduce the effectiveness of the spray. Also, in windy weather the spray could be blown back on you. The best advice is to run with a group of four or more, according to the U.S. Fish and Wildlife Service.

"Running in Oakridge, Oregon, we often have the opportunity to see bears with cubs, elk, and other charismatic megafauna (large, cool animals). I've enjoyed these opportunities when they have arisen but have enough respect for these animals to recognize the potential dangers and am always aware when in their territory," writes trail runner Beverley Anderson-Abs.

Bison

Bison or buffalo can be dangerous any time of year, but the bull male in rut is especially dangerous during mating season in August. Nevertheless, it is best to give bison a wide berth in the backcountry no matter what time of year. Bison attacks entail an aggressive charge followed by an attempt to gore the prey. Most attacks occur near roads or developed areas where the animals roam in their captive habitat in national parks. Privately owned bison ranches exist across North America, but most are fenced and posted with NO TRESPASSING signs.

Like the bison, male elk, moose, and deer can be aggressive during the rut in an effort to protect their harem or prospective mate, or females in the springtime when they are protecting their young. It is best to steer clear of areas frequented by these animals during mating and calving seasons.

Skunks

Another animal to steer clear of no matter what the season is the skunk. Although skunks are mainly out at night, there is always the possibility of a daylight encounter. Most close encounters will result in the skunk spraying a pungent liquid over everything within a 7- to 10-foot radius. However, if there is moisture in the air, the spray can become airborne and travel a much greater distance.

If you have the misfortune of being sprayed by a skunk, try bathing yourself and your clothes in tomato juice. Plan to spend at least one hour soaking and scrubbing to remove the offensive odor, then follow up with a soap-and-water scrub to remove the tomato juice coloring and vegetable smell. Other remedies include vanilla extract (approximately two cups in 1 gallon of water), douche products (for the high vinegar content), or baking soda mixed with hydrogen peroxide or soap.

Mountain Lions

During a 50K trail race on California's Mount Diablo in the fall of 2000, several of the frontrunners spotted a mountain lion, aka cougar, puma, or panther. In the summer of 1993 a mountain lion jumped onto Pikes Peak's well-traveled Barr Trail within 20 feet of an approaching (albeit startled) runner. In both encounters, these runners avoided a potentially dangerous situation when the lions scampered away into the brush. Other runners haven't been as fortunate.

Mountain lions are most common in western states, including Alaska, but they can also be found in Maine and Florida. Be cautious and aware of your surroundings at all times, and heed the following guidelines set forth by the Mountain Lion Foundation, based in Sacramento, California.

- Always venture into wilderness areas with a companion.

- Don't approach a cougar. Most cougars want to avoid humans. Give a cougar the time and space to steer clear of you.

- Never run past or from a cougar. This may trigger its instinct to chase. Make eye contact. Never turn your back to it. Stand your ground.

- Never bend over or crouch down. Doing so makes humans resemble four-legged animal prey. Crouching down or bending over also makes the neck and back of the head vulnerable.

- If you encounter a cougar, make yourself appear larger, and aggressive. Open your jacket, raise your arms, throw stones, branches, etc., without turning away. Wave raised arms slowly, and speak slowly, firmly, and loudly to disrupt and discourage predatory behavior.

- Try to remain standing to protect head and neck and, if attacked, fight back with whatever is at hand (without turning your back)— people have utilized rocks, jackets, garden tools, tree branches, and even bare hands to turn away cougars.

- Keep any pet on a leash—roaming pets are easy prey for cougars. Verify with the land management agency if pets are allowed on trails prior to taking your pet with you. Some state parks— including all state parks in Colorado—do not allow dogs leashed or otherwise on the trails.

Snakes

Smaller than the puma but no less disturbing are snakes. In the United States, twelve to fifteen people die annually from the bites of various venomous snakes. Although the number of deaths by snakebite are small, any snakebite can pose a serious medical situation.

DesertUSA.com has researched and identified four snakes whose venomous bite can be fatal to humans—the coral snake, the copperhead, the cottonmouth water moccasin, and the rattlesnake. The rattlesnake (genus *Crotalus*) is the only venomous snake native to California, but other venomous snakes make their home in the deserts of the American Southwest.

Rattlesnakes come in sixteen different and distinct varieties. While most of the rattlers are concentrated in the southwestern United States, their habitat extends north, east, and south in diminishing numbers and varieties, so every state in the lower forty-eight has one or more varieties.

According to Steve Thompson, who earned his BS in zoology and has been working with rattlesnakes since 1974, most snakes are inactive animals that depend upon concealment for protection. A rattlesnake in its natural habitat is almost impossible to see when motionless and silent. Do not depend on a rattlesnake to rattle before it strikes. Most rattlesnakes will not rattle unless they are frightened or endangered.

Thompson offers this advice for trail runners:

> Be careful to stay out of heavy cover areas while running in the country. It is better to run along clearer or wider established trails. Because a snake is scared of a runner's movement, it is apt to strike a passing victim. Runners must watch the ground in front of them, and be careful where they sit or rest in rattler country.
>
> If you come across a snake, maintain a safe distance, staying at least a body length away from the snake. A snake can normally strike half its body length, but this could be farther if it is facing downhill. Snakes normally aren't aggressive, but be prepared to retreat if a snake comes toward you; it may only be seeking cover. Keep in mind that all rattlesnakes are venomous, even young snakes. Do not disturb, attempt to handle, or kill any venomous snake. A third of those bitten by snakes were trying to catch, handle, or kill the snake. If you have a choice, leave the snake alone. Any sudden or quick movements may aggravate a snake and it may strike. Don't bother the snake and it most likely won't bother you.

Tim Dallas, of Concord, California, relates a story from a run in the East Bay: "I nearly stepped on a rattlesnake on Shell Ridge, but since it had a squirrel in its mouth, I managed to jump clear before it dropped its dinner and tried to strike me. I often come across rattlesnakes on my runs, especially in the mornings or evenings, but I'm now a 'defensive runner' always watching for hazards on the trail."

Fowl

David Kix Miller discovered trail running while living in northern California and Vancouver and vowed to never return to the doldrums of running on the roads again. He recently moved to the Southeast (Nashville, Tennessee), and, while the area is not quite as glorious, he found that there are actually a number of great places to run trails there. Driven by the heat and humidity, he began pushing his runs later and later into the evening, and as the days of summer fell shorter and shorter he often found himself running his local trails at night. He encouraged his girlfriend to try it, and, after much resistance, she decided to get up about 4:00 one morning and give it a shot.

"So . . . under headlamp, off she headed into the hills that foggy morning. She called me later that day and described the horrifying scene (to her anyway) where she heard a loud thump, thump, thump and then experienced excruciating pain like talons piercing into her head. She said she swatted at the mysterious creature in the dark and flailed around on the ground until the creature went away and she was *never* going to run in the dark again! Of course, I assumed that she probably got hooked up in a tree branch, or crossed paths with a little bird, and I shamelessly accused her of embellishing the story and making a big deal out of nothing. Until, that is, about two weeks later when I was enjoying a nice jaunt along the same trail about 10:00 one night. Coming down from the hills, I noticed that I was gaining on another headlamp about a mile in front of me, and caught the guy just before the trailhead. In the usual 'hey you run out here at night a lot' conversation, he was kind enough to share a friendly warning with me. . . . In separate incidents, two of his friends had been attacked on this very same trail by a *huge* owl a couple of weeks before, one requiring stitches to his scalp!"

David Wise was running on a carriage trail in the Vanderbilt Estate and came upon a flock of turkeys. There were some youngsters in the flock, and apparently the mother was not pleased with his presence. She spread her wings as far as she could and began to amble toward him while making a loud cackling noise. Knowing when he was not welcome, he did an about-face and was not followed.

Insects and Other Pests

Many areas frequented by trail runners are notorious for pesky insects, including those that sting—bees, hornets, wasps, yellowjackets, and scorpions—and those that cause nagging bites, like gnats and mosquitoes. Most stings and bites are more of an annoyance than anything else unless they generate an allergic reaction. Trail runners who suffer from allergies related to stings should carry an appropriate medical kit and wear a Medic Alert bracelet. Allergy shots are an option if stings have caused allergic reactions in the past. The best defenses against insects are to avoid wearing sweet-smelling perfumes or colognes (including hair spray), to tightly seal energy drinks, and to wrap and store any food in a waist pack. It is better to wear white, tan, beige, or light-colored clothing, which does not attract bees. Calamine lotion to combat itching is a great addition to any medical kit.

Ticks

Ticks are divided into soft ticks and hard ticks. The deer tick, a member of the hard tick family, is known to transmit Lyme disease to humans through the bloodstream. Lyme disease is most prevalent in the Northeast and upper Midwest and in northern California and southern Oregon, but it has been reported throughout the country. If left untreated, Lyme disease can cause serious damage and chronic problems to the nervous system or circulatory system.

Tall grasses, wooded areas, and shrubby vegetation often harbor ticks waiting to jump on a passing host. Equipped with grasping forelegs, these bloodsucking parasites find a spot on the host to sink their mouths into and feed. Once they are filled with blood, they drop off the host.

To deter ticks, apply insect repellent before a trip to wooded or grassy areas (some repellents are formulated especially for ticks). Check for ticks after every run. It is easier to spot ticks on light-colored clothing, so dress accordingly. Carefully inspect your bare legs, arms, neck, and ear canals. To remove a tick, use tweezers, grasping hold of the body. Take care to remove all parts of the tick, including the head.

Poison Ivy

Blossoming trees, abundant wildflowers, and moss-covered rocks all provide a distinct beauty to a forest. Less appealing to trail runners is poison ivy. Each year ten to fifty million Americans develop an allergic rash after contact with this weed. Some people do not suffer any adverse reactions even after brushing up against poison ivy leaves, but statistics are not favorable—two out of every three people are prone to an allergic reaction.

Jim Dunphy of Herndon, Virginia, has extensively researched poison ivy and says that it usually grows as a vine twining on tree trunks or straggling over the ground, but the plant often forms upright bushes if it has no support on which it may climb. Only Hawaii, Alaska, and some areas in Nevada are free from poison ivy. Species related to poison ivy include poison oak, which grows in California, the Pacific Northwest, and nearby regions of Canada, and poison sumac, which grows in the eastern United States. Poison oak and poison sumac are shrubs, with the former having three leaflets per stem like poison ivy and the latter having rows of six to ten leaflets. One leaflet is at the end of the stem. The others are in one or more rows opposite one another.

The tissues of all these plants contain a sap somewhat like carbolic acid, called urushiol. This sap is extremely irritating to the skin. An allergic reaction can develop within ten minutes after exposure, and a rash can become visible within twelve to twenty-four hours. Sap may be brushed onto the clothing or skin of anyone coming in contact with the plants or from contact with others, including pets, that have come in contact with the plants, but only if the oil remains on their skin or fur. Eruptions themselves are not a source of infection. Some people are so sensitive to the sap that being near droplets in the air can cause a rash to form and spread over the body.

The worst thing to do after contact with poison ivy is to itch or rub the infected area, since such activity can easily transfer the sap to other areas. Topical agents such as calamine lotion or baking soda compresses can combat the itching caused by a bout with poison ivy. Preventative measures with a pre-rinse like Technu on potentially affected areas may reduce the spread of the rash. Injections for those prone to allergic reactions from poison ivy may warrant consideration.

Trail runner Ron Wolf recommends a double soaping protocol to help prevent the reaction to these irritants. "In the shower (never, ever take a bath after running near these plants), get wet, turn the water off, use soap and scrub up a lot of suds especially on exposed parts (lower legs), then rinse well. Also rinse off the soap bar and your wash towel (or whatever). Then do it again (wet, water off, suds, rinse). I haven't had a reaction since starting to do this. Normal soap works fine. Also, the irritating oils may be in trail dust (especially in the West after the rains stop for the season and things dry out). So best to follow this protocol after every trail run in locations where these plants are found."

Poison ivy flourishes on sandy, stony, or rocky shores of streams, rivers, and lakes, as well as sprouting in thickets along the borders of wooded areas. It is most dangerous in the spring and summer months when sap is fertile and plants tend to bruise easily.

Other Hazardous Plant Life

Stinging nettles, burrs, and cacti have the potential for short-term annoyance to the trail runner. Though the duration of a sting or poke from one of these plants may not be as pronounced or long lasting as that of a bout of poison ivy, such contact can still be extremely irritating. Few remedies are available to combat the immediate effects of an encounter with any one of these plants during a run, except to pick off the menacing stickers. Soap and water applied as soon as possible on and around the affected area mitigates the ache.

In addition to contact with obnoxious weeds and plants, ingestion of poisonous fruits and berries can be hazardous to trail runners. Anyone unable to identify plants and berries that grow in or around particular trail routes should refrain from sampling, since results could be disastrous.

Misadventures

Hal Walter lives and runs in the Wet Mountains near Westcliffe, Colorado.

I find bolts of high-voltage electricity being hurled at me by a guy named Zot far more frightening than stepping on a poisonous serpent or staring down a hungry puma. I should know, I've experienced all three.

The time-honored mountaineer's rule of being off the peak by noon was not instituted so people could get back to town in time for happy hour. In the summer, moisture tends to rise over the mountains in the afternoon, then raise havoc in the form of thunderstorms the rest of the day.

Never one to practice all my preachings, I climbed Venable Peak, 13,333 feet, in Colorado's Sangre de Cristo Mountains one afternoon a few summers ago. It looked safe enough when I started; but when adding my name to the sheet in the jam jar at the summit, I heard a rumble that got my attention. Sure enough, a thunderboomer was heading my way with fury. I ended up getting shelled big time by a driving sheet of hail and taking some big chances to get back down below timberline.

Lightning is electrifying to be sure, but the distinct buzz of a rattlesnake underfoot also gives quite a jolt. For those of you who don't think snakes live in the mountains, I've seen rattlesnakes as high as 8,800 feet near the middle of their latitudinal range in Colorado.

Once while running downhill on one of my favorite mountain trails, I stepped right on the rattles of a buzz worm. The snake instinctively rolled over and snagged me in the midsole of my running sneakers. I stood on the trail shaking with disbelief as the snake slithered away. If I had been walking, it probably would have nailed me square in the ankle. Luckily I was running and my foot was back in the air by the time the snake reacted. If you think you're going to see a snake before you step on it, you better have pretty good eyes. I can pass the driver's test from double the prescribed distance. Only blind luck saved me from this snake's fangs.

I have on occasion seen other rattlers before it was too late. I remember spying one big timber rattler coiled when I was about three steps away. I turned off the trail and watched the snake bob his head exactly three times before striking at the thin air that would have been my ankle. I believe the snake was doing math in his head and counting my steps through vibrations in the ground. No warning rattle or anything. Other snakes have been courteous and have rattled when I got too close. I merely passed around them and left them alone.

The first time I saw a lion on the trail I was convinced that these animals are not something with which you want to do hand-to-hand combat. I rounded a switchback and spooked three mule deer to the uphill side of me. A couple of steps later the oak brush on the downhill side exploded in a tawny blur as the startled lion ran downhill about 30 yards, then stopped and turned broadside. For a few seconds I thought this sighting was pretty darn cool. But when I leaned over and put my hands on my knees to get a better look, the lion took a step toward me. I stood back up and shouted at the lion. It turned and—with no lack of attitude—slowly wandered away. Then I turned and ran away at very high speed. Knowing what I know now, I did some things wrong and some things right. But all in all, I still think it was worth it to have seen that lion.

In fact all of these dangers were worth it. It's the idea that something out there can kill you that makes the experience of trail running truly wild, something beyond putting one foot in front of the other. For me, that is the allure.

PERSONAL SAFETY

The thought of being attacked by a wild animal during a run is frightening indeed, though no more frightening than the threat of being attacked by another person. Although women are more at risk than men, both sexes should follow the safety procedures outlined below by the Road Runners Club of America.

The Road Runners Club of America's General Running Safety Tips

1. DON'T WEAR HEADPHONES. Use your ears to be aware of your surroundings. Your ears may help you avoid dangers your eyes may miss during evening or early morning runs.

2. Carry identification or write your name, phone number, and blood type on the inside sole of your running shoe. Include any medical information.

3. Always stay alert and aware of what's going on around you. The more aware you are, the less vulnerable you are.

4. Carry a cell phone or change for a phone call. Know the locations of call boxes and telephones along your regular route.

5. Trust your intuition about a person or an area. React on your intuition and avoid a person or situation if you're unsure. If something tells you a situation is not "right," it isn't.

6. Alter or vary your running route pattern; run in familiar areas if possible. In unfamiliar areas, such as while traveling, contact a local RRCA club or running store. Know where open businesses or stores are located in case of emergency.

7. Run with a partner. Run with a dog.

8. Write down or leave word of the direction of your run. Tell friends and family of your favorite running routes.

9. Avoid unpopulated areas, deserted streets, and overgrown trails. Avoid unlit areas, especially at night. Run clear of parked cars or bushes.

10. Ignore verbal harassment. Use discretion in acknowledging strangers. Look directly at others and be observant, but keep your distance and keep moving.

11. Run against traffic so you can observe approaching automobiles.

12. Wear reflective material if you must run before dawn or after dark.

13. Practice memorizing license tags or identifying characteristics of strangers.

14. Carry a noisemaker. Get training in self-defense.

15. Look both ways before crossing. Be sure the driver of a car acknowledges your right of way before crossing in front of a vehicle. Obey traffic signals.

16. When using multiuse trails, follow the rules of the road. If you alter your direction, look over your shoulder before crossing the trail to avoid a potential collision with an oncoming cyclist or passing runner.

17. CALL POLICE IMMEDIATELY if something happens to you or someone else, or you notice anyone out of the ordinary. It is important to report incidents immediately.

Road Runners Club of America
1501 Lee Hwy, Suite 140
Arlington, Va 22209

NAVIGATION

Maps and the ability to read them are essential when you are trail running, especially when running in unfamiliar areas. Natural and man-made landmarks are helpful when a map is not handy, but both lose their relevance when darkness or a storm ensues. In remote areas, including a cell phone or GPS instrument in a waist pack can be a lifesaver.

Running with a partner who is familiar with a trail and the surrounding area may reduce the potential for getting lost. Choose someone who runs at a comparable speed or at least someone who will wait at confusing intersections. Remember though, even runners who frequent the same trail over and over can get lost. Runners often marvel at the change in a trail from its leaf-strewn state in autumn to a snow- and ice-covered path in winter. A trail that is run north to south looks quite different when run in the opposite direction, particularly if run at different times during the day or night. If the trail is uphill in one direction, it means downhill in the other direction, thereby providing a completely different appearance and experience.

Trails may also look different on race day, even if the course has been traveled many times during training runs. One reason is that the addition of course markers—from bright-colored neon flagging to large white dots of flour at intersections—alters the look of the trail. Another is that increased leg speed changes stride length, resulting in very different foot plants along the trail.

If you are lost, the best recommendation is to backtrack to a recognized point on the trail, rather than continue down the path into further uncertainty. This is true whether in a race or during a training run. When backtracking, stay on the well-worn path rather than creating new trails that will cause further confusion.

Whether the potential danger affecting a trail runner is related to plant life or wildlife, based on the weather, human error, or a combination thereof, heed whatever advice is available. Above all, use good common sense when dealing with the elements, no matter what they presently are or might become.

Running Partners

Human companions provide encouragement, conversation, and support and are relatively easy to find. A good trail running partner is someone who is compatible with your pace, style of running, schedule, location, and particular running goals. A trail race is an ideal place to start the search for such a companion. Check out local events first because chances are good that entrants live within a more convenient geographic range; then consider regional events. At least one competitor in a race will be running a pace similar to yours, but do not eliminate potential companions who run at a different pace. A comparably paced runner provides companionship throughout a run, a slower runner helps regulate the pace for recovery efforts, whereas the faster runner elevates a workout to a quicker and more challenging standard. Casting a wider net reaps greater returns and a better chance of finding someone who lives or works nearby and has a similar training schedule. Be open to partnering up with runners of all ages. Runners who are forty and over, the masters' age category, can provide as much enjoyment as a partner in their teen years. There are also virtual running partners, or coaches, who may not always run with you, but are at the ready to provide tips on training and racing and can help design a plan appropriate for your level of ability and fitness.

Running club newsletters, specialty running stores, recreation centers, health clubs, fitness magazines, and running-related Web sites are additional resources to investigate. Newsletters, magazines, and Web sites list events and activities, whereas running stores often lead workouts from their location or sponsor weekly runs at other venues. Running partners can be found on craigslist and even social networking resources such as Facebook and Twitter. Some sites may not cater specifically to the trail runner but may offer additional ideas, resources, or contacts.

Although many road running clubs have a trail running component in the form of weekly workouts or an organized trail run such as the 3-mile Great Spillway Classic hosted by the New Orleans Track Club, consider joining or starting an organized or informal trail running club that focuses specifically on trail running.

One model comes from Adam Feerst, who started an informal trail running club in the Denver foothills in spring 2000 that has since achieved great success. The impetus for the club grew from Feerst's love of trail running, his desire to share his passion with others, and to travel as a group to mountain races. At the first posted workout, four people showed up. Attendance dipped to just one the following week and then slowly grew to a high turnout of twenty-five the first year. Weekly runs now average thirty to fifty people during the summer and ten to twenty through the winter. The runs are open to runners of all ages and abilities, there are no annual membership dues, and the atmosphere is friendly and supportive. Each run has a variety of different route options, so runners of different speeds can all start and finish together. Group leaders—there are about seven—post runs on Yahoo Groups (they have expanded to Facebook and Twitter and redesigned the denvertrail runners.org site), where the group has an e-mail list of over 1,800. The Web site has route maps and other info about the group. "I have made a big effort to organize the group and Web site to make it as inviting and easy to use as possible," says Feerst. "I get tremendous joy sharing my passion for trail running with others. I hope I've turned a lot of people on to the sport and exposed many to trails they didn't know existed. An added bonus is making new friends. More than a few relationships have spawned and jobs have been found through the group."

California's Dirt Dogs Trail Club based in the East Bay has weekly runs with an established practice of trail marking its courses. This group, founded in 1999, rotates its trail running location weekly and posts it to club members via e-mail. The club designates a trail marker who carries flour in a specially designed plastic bottle with holes in the right diameter for a crisp, clean arrow that uses a minimal amount of flour so the trail marker can easily carry it along the course. The sweeper, who carries a whisk broom, can brush away the markings in a couple of quick strokes. "We find this practice of marking—and removing the markings—keeps the rangers in our districts happy and is environmentally friendly. There is also the issue of responsibility for the organizers which is satisfied by the sweeper who makes sure there are no injured or disoriented runners still out on the course," says club member Dave Peck.

Another option for trail runners to consider is attending a camp or a trail running vacation—either domestically or internationally. One model in the United States comes from Terry Chiplin, founder of Active at Altitude in Estes Park, Colorado. "We wanted to share our excitement in the possibilities that surround us; there are miles of trails in the area, starting from 7,500 feet to over 14,000 feet. So I came up with the concept of trail running camps, with runners staying at our mountain lodge. We provide meals, drinks, workshops and seminars on useful trail running stuff like how to ascend and descend efficiently, what gear to wear, hydration and fuel. I invite guest speakers from the amazing array of local talent and expertise. Now I love running these trails; the experience becomes even more special when you can share these joys with like-minded people. Running trails connect people with being alive—there is so much in our society that is repetitive and boring; trails connect us with the environment, the trees, the animals, the insects, the birds, with the very essence of what being alive truly means. We have had runners attending camps that have had life-changing realizations being here. We now hold trail running camps several times a year—the climate here in Estes Park means we can run trails pretty much all year-round. Even if snow does stick around, we can snowshoe instead. The camps are intimate, no more than fifteen runners, and offer great value and an opportunity to run trails and learn from experienced trail runners in one of the most beautiful places for training anywhere in the world."

Some tour groups are starting trail running vacations to international destinations that may be coupled with a race or event. These are usually fairly small groups of eight to fifteen participants and go to traditional as well as more exotic locales.

RUNNING WITH KIDS

Sometimes a trail running partner is as close as a family member. Even if a future trail runner is added to your family through the birth of a child, the advent of all-terrain strollers (see Chapter 7 on equipment) has allowed parents to bring children with them on their trail runs. Make sure the child is old enough to hold her or his head steady, especially if the trail run is likely to be turbulent. Make sure the little one has plenty of padding and warm clothes. A blanket is always a good idea as well. Not all trails are baby jogger–friendly. Look for smoother surfaces and always make sure the passenger is enjoying the ride. It is better to do shorter loops, just in case a quick return home is warranted.

When using a stroller on the trail, be considerate of other runners, especially when running with a group. In many cases, it is best to leave the all-terrain stroller at home. Taking a fast trail hike using a front or backpack child carrier is a friendly alternative. After introducing the little one to workouts via the stroller or pack, chances are good that a trail aficionado will eventually emerge and become a future running partner.

RUNNING WITH DOGS

Bipeds make great partners on the trail, but don't discount our four-footed friends. Dogs provide an advantage over human partners because they can carry gear, and they may see, smell, or hear things that humans cannot. Like humans, they provide companionship as they share the trail running experience. However, dogs can be hard to encourage, often prove disruptive to other trail users, might do environmental and trail damage, or may require modifications to pace or a change to a scheduled workout due to fatigue or stubbornness. Plus they require extra care, attention, and money.

Dogs are like people: Some want to sit around and eat, while others prefer getting out in the hills for a workout. Since they can't communicate with words, evaluate other signs relayed by your dog to determine if trail running is really something he or she considers as much fun as you do.

Known as man's best friend, a dog can also be a trail runner's most faithful companion. However, some breeds are more amenable than others to trail running, with weight, size, age, energy level, and temperament being determining factors. The environment, type of terrain, trail location, and duration of the run further influence the choice and narrow the search.

While a mature 80-pound hound may be comfortable during a cool, short thirty-minute loop, a two-hour run in the heat and humidity could devastate such a canine. The younger (two- to five-year-old) and smaller (30- to 45-pound) pooch usually has better endurance and speed, but the excitability of certain breeds requires lots of workout time. Robert DeFranco, a certified canine behavior counselor, says, "All dogs can benefit from a reasonable running exercise program. Depending on the breed, some dogs can handle a run of longer duration better than others. For example, a breed that was bred for running or fieldwork, such as a lab or a golden retriever, can probably handle more than a small, short-legged dog such as a dachshund or a short-nosed breed such as a bulldog or pug."

Dog trainer and certified behaviorist Tim Mullally adds, "Look at the breed's intended use, and climate of its origin. For example, Dalmatians are bred as carriage dogs in Egypt, hence they can handle long-distance running in hotter climates. The Siberian husky is bred for long-distance running in northern, harsh climates, and Dobermans are also bred for long-distance running. For rougher trails consider a slightly bigger-boned bloodline like an Akita, which is bred for bear hunting in the mountains of Japan. Most hunting dogs and herding breeds will also be good choices. The best thing to do is to research the breed, look at the job at hand for the dog, and use a little common sense."

Any preexisting condition, along with the health of the dog's hips, muscles, and joints, should be reviewed by a veterinarian before starting a canine on a running program. After receiving a clean bill of health, start the dog with short jogs (lasting no more than thirty minutes), and increase distance training over time. DeFranco adds, "I usually recommend starting dogs that are younger, middle-aged, or overweight on a moderate program of walking or jogging for ten to fifteen minutes a day, increasing to twice a day in a few weeks. Male or female, neutered or not, makes no difference when it comes to exercise; but monitor for signs of fatigue and adjust training accordingly."

"Pounding on the ground is too much for a young dog," says Karen Peak, of Prince William County, Virginia, owner of West Wind Dog Training, who has been working with dogs since 1982. "Don't start trail running with a dog until he/she is fully physically mature—upward growth is complete for most breeds in one year, but some breeds will continue to 'mature' until they are two to three years old. A dog may physically look like they can run, but they might not be ready. You can start training and working with a young dog to hone behaviors, but don't start running with your dog until he/she is older. Before you start running with your dog, have a full vet physical to include X-rays of the hips, elbows, and knees. Ensure there are no elbow issues, no luxating patellas (kneecap not tracking correctly), and no hip dysplasia."

Always keep a dog leashed, especially in wilderness areas where a pet may come in contact with other wildlife and activate predatory instincts on the part of the feral species. Obey posted signs and refrain from taking a dog into areas posted off limits. Supplement all leash training with voice commands, and consider including a series of dog obedience classes in the training program.

Running is natural for most dogs, and tails wag in readiness for a run as soon as the leash is attached to the collar. Since a dog is unable to discuss fitness level and ability, and most dogs have no concept of pace, the owner must watch for signs of fatigue during every run. Don't wait until a dog gravitates to the nearest tree, lies down panting, and refuses to move before realizing the distance was too great for the dog to endure. Heat and humidity can be a dangerous combination for dogs that are pushed too far or too fast. Dogs sweat through the pads on their feet and do not release heat as efficiently as humans do, so they can easily overheat. Dogs need to replenish their fluid levels as they exercise, and if no water exists on the trails, be sure to carry additional water.

Be aware of trail hazards that can affect a dog's ability to run. Burrs, thorns, cacti, and nettles can easily become imbedded in a dog's paw. Sharp rocks, gravel, sticks, and ice can cause lesions that result in red, swollen pads. Dogs, like humans, can develop overuse injuries and chronic knee, leg, or shoulder pain from overtraining. Always watch a dog's movement for signs of muscle soreness and fatigue. After running with a dog, inspect its fur, paws, and inside the ears for ticks and burrs, and pads for swelling and redness.

Kysmit, My Canine Running Companion

By Jill Suzanne Sparks

In May 2009 I lost my running partner. For twelve years he had run by my side—from the rugged coast of British Columbia, to the frozen Canadian Arctic, to the sweltering sandy desert trails of New Mexico. Together we had run them all. His name was Kysmit. And he was my dog.

Born to run long, Kysmit was a Siberian husky. At eight months old Kysmit's energy requirements were no longer satisfied by long walks. He needed more. So, like any new runner, Kysmit started slowly and added distance gradually to his weekly runs. I remember that when Kysmit was a pup, running the mountains of Vancouver Island with me, he was too small to make the steep climbs. I often had to support his back legs and hoist him up. At the end of the trail, he would rest under a tree in the shade, a smile spread across his face.

Huskies are known for their wandering spirits, and Kysmit had a double dose of it. "This time, he won't run away," I'd tell myself. And without fail he would tear down the trail in front of me, catch a glimpse of a furry friend in the forest, and be off. So for the first seven years of his life, Kysmit ran on a leash. Running dogs with a harness system is a good idea. Being a natural "puller" I avoided the harness with Kysmit and simply ran him on his collar with a light long leash (I used a 10-foot piece of thin climbing rope). During technical sections, climbs, or descents, I simply let go of this leash. This allowed him and me to run these sections safely, but just in case a furry friend caught his eye, I could easily step on his long leash and have control again. Many runners tie their dog's leash around their waist. On the trail this is dangerous. The dog could easily pull you off balance, ending in a fall that could hurt both of you. Retractable leashes can also be a hazard as they tangle easily.

While running a secluded trail in Colorado, Kysmit nearly dragged me up a mountainside. He was barking and growling; I had never seen such behavior from him. After much commotion and luring him down the trail with the Power Bones (dog energy bars) I always carried in my pocket, I discovered the cause of his behavior. High above us, a mountain lion was stalking two deer. Being leashed saved him from harm. Of course, as Kysmit became more experienced on the trail and realized he needed to expend his energy carefully (not run away), I started to let him off leash on remote trails. Running a snow-covered southern Ontario trail one morning in early spring, I learned why the leash is essential. Twelve kilometers from the trailhead Kysmit and I met up with a sleepy porcupine. After pulling over thirty quills from his front paw and inside of his mouth, I attached his leash once again. In total I pulled over sixty quills from him that day. It was a long time before he was allowed off leash again.

Winter was the best time to run Kysmit, because he was a husky. His best running years were the three we lived in the high Canadian Arctic. Even in minus-40 degree weather he thrived. I bought him booties to protect his feet, but he refused to wear them. When I could not run due to the freezing temperatures, Kysmit ran beside the snowmobile. He logged lots of mileage in the Arctic. In contrast, he loved chasing geckos on our desert vacation runs. Running in those dry, hot conditions he required a lot of special care. His runs were kept shorter and started earlier in the day or later in the evening, and we selected routes that had water access points. Nevertheless I always carried a bottle for him. As a pup he had learned to drink from a water bottle and bladder. Most breeds will run till they drop, so you need to respect your dog's limits in all conditions.

Kysmit loved to run. He never needed encouragement to hit the trail, and more than once swayed me with his big brown eyes to tie up my laces. I could never seem to deny him the joy of a trail run. And I shared this joy. Running beside my canine partner afforded me solitude, yet his presence gave me the pleasure of having companionship on the trail. We shared the beauty and serenity together. Often at the top of a climb or high up on a ridge, he would pause, drinking in the view. The magnificence of our surroundings never passed him by.

Later in life when his arthritis became too painful for him to run, we hiked the trails together. The trail perked him up, and momentarily he seemed to forget his pain. At times, when a squirrel caught his eye or a log crossed our path, he would take off again. But these moments were fleeting toward the end. And what once brought him such joy, he had to give up.

Kysmit and I had a special bond that only comes from running with someone. It didn't matter that he was a dog. The joy trail running gave him was the same it brought me. As I run our familiar trails together now with my new canine partner, I often smile in memory of our many runs and years together.

RUNNING WITH BURROS, HORSES, AND MORE

Another animal considered by some to be an excellent training companion is a burro. Individuals who run with burros are primarily those who train to compete in races hosted by the Western Pack Burro Association. Pack burro racing is the only sport known to be indigenous to Colorado, and it is one that is taken most seriously by those who do it.

Veteran burro racer Hal Walter relates the following: "The sport demands a high level of fitness from both human and beast, as well as some peculiar talents. These animals see little glory in running 20 to 30 miles, and it requires considerable skill to persuade them through a course generally routed over terrain strewn with boulders, snowfields, talus, and rock glaciers. The animal is equipped with a 15-foot lead rope and a packsaddle weighted with mining gear. This sport requires serious physical fitness on the part of both human and animal. It's more like a cross between a horse race and a mountain marathon."

Burro racing and handling is not for everyone. Considerable time and effort is required to train burros to run alongside a runner, not to mention the cost and acreage necessary for the burro's upkeep.

Another organized trail event where animals and humans compete together is Ride & Tie. A Ride & Tie team is composed of two people and one horse. One person starts out on foot while the other is riding.

At a strategic distance the rider dismounts, ties the horse to (usually) a tree, and continues down the trail on foot. The person who started on foot eventually reaches the horse, mounts, and rides to catch his or her partner, where they will exchange, or continue farther ahead and tie the horse. This "leapfrog" technique is repeated over the entire course ranging from 10 to 40 miles.

Laura Christofk, an avid fan of Ride & Tie explains: "The Ride & Tie horse is a completely integrated part of the team. Veteran Ride & Tie horses understand how the game is played and truly enjoy the camaraderie of their teammates and the competition with others. Race strategy considers all three partners' strengths and weaknesses to maximize the team's abilities, with the priority being the safety and physical well-being of the equine.

"Close friendships develop through Ride & Ties between partners as well as with other competitors. Ride & Ties are typically very challenging and pit everyone against the trail and weather, not merely each other."

Only a very few organized events include llama competition, but this animal makes an excellent training partner for some people. Llamas are known for their sure footing and strength and have been long revered as excellent pack carriers whose two-toed, soft-padded feet don't damage the environment the way hooves or hiking boots do. According to Tom Sobal, who has raced a llama or two, the breed is not very fast, certainly not as fast as a burro. In fact, Sobal says he and his burro Maynard clocked a 4:50 mile, whereas a llama he trained with only managed a 5:25 for the same distance. Since llamas are part of the camel family, they tend to spit as a way of communicating with other animals in the herd. However, humans are usually targeted with expectoration only when the llamas are scared, feel threatened, or have been mistreated.

"Running with another animal that is bigger, stronger, and/or faster allows a runner the opportunity to make that animal carry the extra load of water, clothing, gear, or food. This lets the runner move freely without the burden of added weight and packs. The carrier of gear can also be another human—a practice known as 'muling,'" says Sobal.

CHAPTER 12

Caring for the Trail

Whether a trail is a new addition to an area, a long-established component of a citywide park system, or a remote animal pathway, trail use should be considered a privilege and not a right. As trail users, runners should be respectful of their precious natural resources and do what they can to ensure that trails last well into the future. There are numerous advocacy and stewardship programs for the trail runner to consider, and if one doesn't exist in your area, consider starting one to preserve and maintain trails.

MULTIUSE

Regardless if a trail runner enjoys an area alone or with a partner, multiuse issues should be understood and addressed. Two primary categories of trail users exist: nonmotorized, including backpackers, hikers, equestrians, mountain bikers, and trail runners; and motorized, including dirt bikers, all-terrain vehicles (ATVs), and off-highway vehicles (OHVs). Trail systems within national parks or recreation areas often ban certain modes of transportation—usually the motorized variety—but some areas prohibit mountain bikes, equestrians, and trail runners as well. Areas may restrict trail access on occasion due to environmental concerns, wildlife issues, or natural hazards.

Sometimes trails, though open to the public, are closed to trail running events. Should an event be denied access to an area, find out why. Perhaps the reason for restricting access is due to limited knowledge about the sport. Use a positive approach when meeting with appropriate authorities and present educational brochures and flyers describing the positive benefits of trail running. Share information and work with organizations instead of against them.

If an area is posted with NO TRESPASSING signs, refrain from using the trail, and always seek permission to use trails located on private land. Further, if a trail marker indicates a particular route, don't deviate or create meandering social trails (also dubbed spider trails)—always stay on the marked path. In areas that require a user fee—typically for parking but may include trail use as well—do not cut a rope or bypass a tollbooth to escape payment.

ENVIRONMENTALISM

Experiencing the natural sights, sounds, smells, and surfaces found on trails is a huge part of the desire to run trails, as opposed to roads. A high density of too many trails in certain areas detracts from this appeal. Trails have a negative impact on the natural environment they pass though. With a growing population, increased trail use, and recognition that natural areas cannot be all things for all people, trail use may become more restricted in the future. Thus the number, type, and amount of trails, and their use, are and will be limited in certain areas in order to preserve the environment, protect resources, and retain the quality experience all trail users seek. Trails will likely become a limited resource in the future, and trail runners will have an advantage because of the flexibility to adapt to all types of trails.

On trails that allow participation by all groups, cooperation is the key to peaceful coexistence, and it is imperative to ensure the trail will always be around to enjoy. Although each user group enjoys an activity that may be quite different from another's form of recreation, preservation and respect for the environment should be the shared concern of all users. Most users have an advocacy group to turn to for education and support. For example, the International Mountain Bicycling Association (IMBA), headquartered in Boulder, Colorado, is a nonprofit organization whose mission is to promote mountain bicycling opportunities that are environmentally sound and socially responsible. The association encourages low-impact riding, volunteer trail work participation, cooperation among different trail user groups, and innovative trail management solutions.

Trail groups are adopting and publicizing rules for responsible trail use as they relate to a particular region. But many of the rules are relevant to other trails as well and can be applied to them with minor modifications. A good template is provided by the Contra Costa Canal Regional Trails:

- Be safe, considerate, and aware of your impact on the trail and other trail users.

- For everyone's safety, keep to the right. Proceed single file around blind curves.

- For your safety, headphones are not advised.

- Dogs must be on leash where posted, and under full verbal control elsewhere. Please clean up after your dog.

User groups can work together to practice environmental and social responsibility for the benefit of trail systems through numerous conservation efforts. Schedule work days to repair, maintain, preserve, and improve trails. Work days can be organized through an existing nonprofit group or volunteer association with support from a local forest service department, a park system, or a recreation area. All trail users should be encouraged to participate in work days. Publish a list of trail work days in the local newspaper, on Web sites, at races, and at club events. Reach out to the numerous and varied users of trails for support.

Additional stewardship methods include adoption and fund-raising. Identify particular trails and set up an adopt-a-trail program that includes annual trail maintenance, repair, and cleanup. Organize fund-raising efforts at races. Set up an information booth and distribute literature on trail systems, and seek donations. Include a check-off box on race entry forms designating funds to trail maintenance projects.

Offer educational trail safety programs that can be jointly set up to benefit many user groups. IMBA offers a mountain bike patrol service that can be implemented by other user groups. Be creative and start a program with ATV or dirt bike owners to monitor trail systems in specific areas. Include land managers and policymakers when developing programs. Local retailers, manufacturers, and corporate representatives may support your cause through sponsorship.

Many national organizations provide direction for outdoor recreation, including Leave No Trace, Inc. The LNT principles of outdoor ethics form the framework of their message and include the following:

- Plan ahead and prepare.

- Travel on durable surfaces.

- Dispose of waste properly.

- Leave what you find.

- Respect wildlife.

- Be considerate of other visitors.

ATRA promotes the following responsible trail runner tips compiled by longtime ATRA board member Tom Sobal:

- Stay on marked and existing trails.

- Don't cut switchbacks.

- Go through puddles, not around them.

- Climb or jump over fallen trees instead of going around them.

- When multiple trails exist, run on the one most worn.

- Do not litter, leave no trace, and pack everything out you packed in.

- Use minimum-impact techniques to dispose of human waste.

- Leave what you find—take only photographs.

- Close all gates that you open.

- Keep pets leashed at all times, and be sure to leave pets at home when running in areas posted "no pets."

- Stop to help others in need: Even while racing, sacrifice your event to aid other trail users who might be in trouble.

- Volunteer at trail races—before, during, or after an event.

- Volunteer, support, and encourage others to participate in trail maintenance days.

- Do not disturb or harass wildlife or livestock.

- Stay off closed trails and obey all posted regulations.

- Respect private property; get permission first to go on private land.

- Do not run on muddy or very dusty trails; pick another route so that you don't further damage the trail and cause unnecessary erosion.

- Warn other trail users when passing from behind by calling out "hello" or "trail" well in advance to avoid startling them.

- Know the area you plan to run in and let at least one other person know where you intend going.

- Dress for the conditions—both existing and potentially changeable.

- Carry plenty of water.

- Be ready to yield to other trail users (bikers, hikers, equestrians).

- Uphill runners yield to downhill runners.

- When preparing to pass a runner, yell "trail" well in advance.

- Know your limits.

This list has been further refined as a *Rules on the Run* document available at www.trailrunner.com in a .pdf version.

The basis for every outdoor experience rests in safety, appreciation, and environmental awareness. Enjoy trail runs with this in mind.

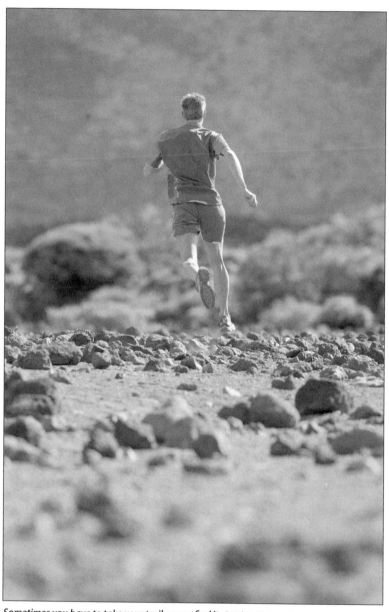

Sometimes you have to take your trail as you find it. Stephan/Gripmaster

CHAPTER 13

Racing and Directing a Race

The number of trail races in the United States has grown significantly during the past decade from approximately 450 events in 1994 to well over 1,000 in 2009. New trail races, many of which are part of a series of trail races, are cropping up each year to meet the demands of runners, from recreational participants to the competitive athlete. Events range in distance from 1-mile fun runs for children to 100-plus miles of ultra endurance running, with the majority of races accounted for by ATRA in their annual online events calendar ranging from 5 to 15 miles.

This chapter describes the fundamentals of directing a trail race, including tips and techniques for making trail races more successful and environmentally and runner-friendly, and will offer guidance on selecting a trail race that is right for you. Existing and prospective race directors will learn procedures necessary to stage a well-run trail event from choosing a site and securing a permit to sweeping the course after the race, while improving those tools and skills they already possess. Participants will become more familiar with important elements that every trail race should provide to its registrants and be better prepared to ask the right questions the next time they consider entering a trail race. Without a doubt, this chapter will help trail race newbies and veterans alike have a greater appreciation for the effort that goes into staging a well-run trail race.

ENTERING A TRAIL RACE

Trail racing adds another dimension to the trail running experience. Racing provides an opportunity to visit new areas, explore new trails, run with people of varied ages and ability levels, and enjoy aid stations manned by supportive volunteers. Competition is inherent in racing, but it is not mandatory to run fast—unless of course there are cutoff times imposed by the race, in which case you should use the cutoff time as an incentive to increase training pace in preparation for the event.

Publications including local, regional, and national running magazines and running-related Web sites provide a listing of trail races, though some calendars are more complete than others. Check with specialty running stores or area running clubs for help finding a trail race that is right for you. When choosing a race, either select one that mirrors the terrain and distance of your training program or alter your training to reflect the conditions of the race. The race should provide at least the basics, including a well-marked course, a map and profile of the course, aid on the course where designated on the map (depending on the distance of the race, it may be prudent to carry additional water and food), and accurate timing and results. There should be a contact number, e-mail, or Web site to refer to for additional information before, during, and after the event.

RACE DIRECTOR RESPONSIBILITIES

The race director's job, in addition to choosing the best site and course for an event, is to provide a safe arena for competition and offer participants a positive and memorable experience. This is often a daunting task for a first-time director because of the many uncertainties involved in the process and the steepness of the learning curve. Add to that the potentially severe consequences of an error and the job ahead looms huge. Fortunately, a motivated and enthusiastic individual can become a capable director and make the organization process much smoother if he or she is open to suggestions and seeks input from others experienced in the field.

Some trail race directors make their living from organizing events. But most do not. In order to make a living from organizing trail races, one must administer quality events with good sponsorship support. It is rare that a single trail event will produce enough income for an annual livable salary, mainly because the money from registration fees typically goes toward offsetting expenses. If another source of income for your event is not present in the form of sponsorship dollars, product support, grants, or merchandise sales, the financial cushion could be quite thin. Most companies are more inclined to provide product support rather than cash. If, however, the event benefits a cause or charity, sponsors may be more inclined to invest cash into the race. In short, before committing to a career as a trail race director, closely review a detailed budget to evaluate whether your financial needs and personal goals can be met by organizing one or more events.

It is very common to see trail races that are organized by volunteers through a running group or charitable entity. Volunteer groups hoping to organize a trail race should consider the benefits of budgeting to hire a paid race director. A professional will provide the necessary experience and leadership to better ensure a successful, high-quality event. Contact a local running club or store in your area for some contact names or advertise the position in a local or regional running publication.

Some events have taken the step of incorporating a specific race as part of an employee's job description. Suzanne Mittenthal is the founding director of the Hoosiers Hiking Council, and as part of her job she directs the Tecumseh Trail Marathon, which celebrated its seventh running in December 2009. But regardless of whether the director is paid or is a volunteer, there are certain traits that are important to the job's successful completion.

The successful race director must be organized and detail oriented. Many of the best race directors are those who have run in trail races themselves and have learned from firsthand experience what works and what doesn't. During the course of one's race-directing tenure, it is good practice to either watch, volunteer, or participate in other events to see what other race directors are doing, both good and bad. Borrow ideas that work and scrap those that do not.

In order to do the job well, a race director must be a quick thinker in inevitable, unpredictable, and often complex situations. Nothing ever goes exactly as planned. On arriving at the start line you may find that half the volunteers never checked in for duty, an overnight rainstorm may have washed out part of your course, or the portable toilets may be out of toilet paper. The best advice is to expect the worst, hope for the best, and be prepared for any situation.

Another all-important trait is the ability to effectively delegate responsibilities. Keep in mind, any race is only as strong as its weakest area; hence the director needs to keep tabs on every part of the race. But don't become a micromanager. No one person can do it all. The backbone of any race is its organizing committee, and most likely a large number of volunteers will be in those positions. Never take those volunteers for granted. Offer praise when praise is due, and convey many, many thanks along the way. It is imperative that a race director select excellent people for key support staff and be willing to allow the appointed individuals to manage the various responsibilities they have been assigned.

According to race director Dale Tuck: "If you give someone a task, delegate it completely. Check with them to see if they need help, but do not interfere with their control." The best way to follow up with committee members is to request reports and updates during weekly or monthly meetings.

Patience is probably the one quality possessed by the best race directors. Bob Rosso has been in the business since the 1970s and agrees: "If you have thin skin, forget it. Most runners show great appreciation, but there are always a few who will try your patience." Remember that the director is the point person before, during, and after the event—the one to field all phone calls and e-mails pre- and post-race (unless someone else is designated that task). Be prepared for some outlandish requests prior to the race and both positive and negative comments post-event. During the race, your coat will be the one that is constantly tugged at by runners with a last-minute request. And no matter what is done for the runners, someone will have advice on how it could have been done better. Tuck adds, "By and large, everything that goes right will be claimed by others and everything that goes wrong will be the race director's fault. Of course, if you do screw up, admit it and apologize."

COURSE SELECTION

Once committed to organizing a trail race, the director must select the date, time, and place to stage the event. In choosing a date, consult with area and regional running clubs and check multisport calendars to see what other potentially competing events are slated near or on the same date. Although any race will invariably compete with some other event happening in a particular area on the same weekend, it is worth the effort to select a date when attendance can best be maximized from the targeted market—the trail runner. If another trail race is already slated for the weekend of choice, it would be best to select another date, unless your region is heavily weighted with runners who enjoy doing a race on both Saturday and Sunday. On the other hand, if your trail race is a short race, and the competing race is a long one, the two races may draw from two separate markets such that both events can be staged on the same weekend—one catering to the ultra, the other to the non-ultra crowd. However, the best option is to combine the events. According to East Coast event director Jerry Stage, "Trail running is too good to be kept a secret." Stage encourages neophyte runners at his event as well as seasoned veterans. He added a sampler event to his main event many years ago in an effort to provide entertainment for spouses, kids, and friends who wanted in on activities (picnic and all) but couldn't do the longer run. The shorter race has attracted more local runners to the festivities than might otherwise have come to the event.

The distance selected for a race may be predetermined by the location of the course. One can be creative by doing double and triple loops to gain extra distance, or make an out-and-back route to shorten the course. Whatever style is selected, it will most likely fall into one of the following categories: loop, keyhole or lollipop (where runners head out on one trail, make a large loop, then rejoin the original trail to the finish), out and back, or point to point. When determining the type of course, consider some of the following variables: Will the start/finish area be the same? If not, will it be necessary to provide buses or another mode of shuttling runners to and from the start and finish points? This can be a major expense. Consider the Pikes Peak Ascent, where competitors run from the town of Manitou Springs, Colorado, approximately 13 miles to the 14,115-foot summit of Pikes Peak. There are only two ways back to the start: run or walk down the same trail ascended, or get motorized transport off the mountain. The race committee spends approximately $16,000 (up from a budget of $4,000 in the year 2000) for transportation to get runners back to the start line. If the budget cannot accommodate that kind of expense, better rethink the course.

When choosing a keyhole, lollipop, or out-and-back course, consider the width of the trail and the number of runners it will accommodate so that bottlenecks can be avoided when the field doubles back on itself. If the trail is 3 feet wide, having more than one runner abreast on the trail will prove difficult. But to provide passing zones brings up issues with any permits obtained—in many cases, running off designated trails is forbidden because the practice wreaks havoc with existing ecosystems flanking the trails. No matter what widths are ultimately determined for the route, it is always advisable to provide a wider area at the start point to spread runners out before they reach a singletrack or narrowed trail. Race director Larry Miller, who organizes a four-race cross-country series each fall in the Pikes Peak region of Colorado, has one of the events start on a school track. The runners start with one lap on the track before they head through a gate that opens onto a vast city park with miles of trails. The inside of the track provides a great staging area for the runners, and the school has more than adequate parking nearby.

Parking can often be a huge issue. Scout the location and determine if ample parking exists near the start/finish line. If entrants must pay to park, advise them of that in the entry materials. A great idea from Tom Sobal, who used to organize the Turquoise Lake 20K in Leadville, Colorado, was to provide a cash incentive to runners carpooling with three or more to the start line. Sobal also allowed these energy-conscious athletes to park in the lot closest to the start area. At other events, runners congregate in a staging area and then run together to the start line for a warm-up jog. If a separate staging area is located some distance from the start line, be sure toilets (portable or otherwise) are accessible for runners and an area is provided to leave sweats after completing a warm-up. Another alternative is to offer drop bags to runners when they pick up their packet on race morning.

MEASURING AND MARKING THE COURSE

Assume now that the course has been selected and a preliminary scouting trip has been made. How runable is the route and can it be accurately measured? Are there natural obstacles on the course now, and what future obstacles may require a change in the route prior to race day?

For example, the course may be flanked on either side by large boulders surrounded by loose rock, dirt, and shale. Significant rainfall prior to the event might cause the boulders to become dislodged and fall onto the course. Is there a backup plan to reroute the course? What contingency plans exist for adverse weather? Waiting until race day to make alternate plans is rarely successful because something else always seems to go wrong on race day that requires immediate attention.

A Jones/Oerth Counter (a special type of digital counter named after its inventor Alan Jones and current producer/distributor Paul Oerth) attaches to the front wheel of a bicycle and is a very accurate way to measure the proposed course, but a calibrated computer directly mounted to a mountain bike can also perform the task quite well. Topographical maps are also beneficial in assessing the distance, especially in more remote and hard-to-access areas. If part of the course is in a state or national park, trail distances may have already been measured and documented. Using GPS for marking and measuring courses has become more commonplace. Be sure you calibrate your GPS for accuracy before measuring a course.

However the course is measured, make sure runners are provided with accurate distances so they can anticipate the amount of time they will be out on the course and plan accordingly. Often runners must rely solely on the race director's measuring techniques. Since trail race distances do not readily translate from course to course as they typically do in road events, attempt to provide a detailed and accurate course description (including the elevation changes on the course) in the race entry information. Experienced trail racers can then determine their approximate finish time. When producing race entry information for subsequent year events, provide course records and average finish times for reference.

Trail races are not known for placing mile or kilometer markers on courses. Some runners suggest this as a good practice for considering their pace or progress on a course. The Pikes Peak Ascent and Marathon place markers at every mile on the Barr Trail, and runners have appreciated this effort of the race staff, even though a runner's mile pace varies greatly throughout this particular racecourse—like that of many mountain courses.

USATF in 2008 compiled a list of suggested guidelines for trail marking of ultradistance trail races, and many if not all of these suggestions apply to shorter distance events. The course may be marked with directional signs, flour-marked arrows, bright ecological paper flagging, ribbon, or tape. The chosen color should clearly stand out from the background and be visible to all competitors. For night races, glow sticks or reflectors are a good addition.

Flour, à la Hash House Harriers, is often the preferred method of marking a course, since it dissolves after a few rainfalls. On the other hand, significant foot traffic (or rain) may remove a directional flour arrow before the last runner makes the requisite turn. When selecting flagging, consider one of three options. Place the flagging at eye level every 100 to 200 feet, more frequently if turnoff points occur along the trail. Additional signage with arrows indicating turns is also helpful. The second option is to place flags in the ground. The third option is a combination of the two. All flagging should be of a highly visible neon color. In race entry materials, inform competitors of the type and color of the flagging used to mark the trail and how often it will be found along the course.

Ultrarunner Mark Godale relates the following: "I got lost during a 50K trail race that was marked with red streamers hanging from the trees. Since I am color-blind I can't differentiate between reds and greens, but I didn't know the course was marked with the red streamers until after the race started."

Some race directors neglect to mark their course if it appears obvious that no wrong turn can possibly be made. However, runners like to be reassured they are on course even if it means over-marking the trail in some areas. "Most trail runners have concerns about getting lost," observes race director Mort Nace. "I think that individual navigation should be part of trail running but a race director needs to find a middle ground between keeping the course somewhat wild yet relatively easy for the novice to follow."

"I ran a 10K mountain race in Slovenia that was marked start to finish with uncut yellow tape on either side of the trail. That's 12 miles of tape. I never got lost," says Rickey Gates.

Volunteers standing in place are probably the best course directional markers, although there are often areas in longer distance trail races that are not very accessible, so the prospect of seeing a person on certain portions of a course in a 100-miler is as remote as the terrain may be. If you do use volunteers as "signposts," spend some time instructing them where and how to point a runner in the right direction and provide them with a map of the course before sending them on their way. Many a volunteer has been sent out to a point on a trail course without proper instructions as to his or her duties, and consequently a runner is sent off course.

Carl Sniffen's preferred course marking is, "the person in front of me who knows the route." There are many stories about runners who follow the person in front of them only to get hopelessly lost.

This author was running a race in Japan, came to a junction, and decided to follow the Japanese runner in front of her since there was no marking on the course and surely someone from the country would know the best trail to take. She continued to follow the Japanese runner—who had no idea where he was going—on a trail that wound through a forest back near the start area some twenty minutes out of the way.

Regardless of your method of course marking, safety should always be the top priority. Plan to provide additional markings for exposed tree roots, large rocks, or other natural unmovable obstacles on the course, especially if they are easy to overlook but are in the runner's direct path. Once a course is set, take some runners out on the route to do a test run. According to athlete-turned-race director Kelvin Broad: "Often as you develop a course you get to know it so well that you don't notice the many pitfalls that may exist on the route. Taking other runners on the course lets you see the course in a new light. Your friends will often see difficulties or potential wrong turns that you have overlooked because you are so familiar with the course."

The course should be rechecked for consistent markings and pitfalls on race day before the starter's gun is fired. All flagging and course markings are best removed following the event during a final course sweep. Provide course sweepers with a backpack in which to place discarded flagging.

ENTRY LIMITS

Another element of directing a race that may be predetermined is the number of runners that may participate in the event. The selected route may be restricted to a certain number of entrants either for safety reasons, permit requirements, race director comfort level, quality of experience for competitors, or a combination of these parameters. Safety considerations often dictate the number of competitors a course can handle. According to Dick Vincent, director of the Escarpment 30K in upstate New York: "We set our limit to adequately support the field over the entire course. There are remote areas on the course and evacuation is not always timely and would greatly stress our safety personnel if we did not limit entries into our event."

Vincent further ensures safety in his race by imposing qualifying standards for the competitors. Likewise, the Skyrunning events require participants in their SkyMarathons to be at least eighteen years old with significant high-altitude experience either as a competitive runner or endurance athlete. As an additional safety factor, Skyrunning events (among others) require that all registered runners check in on race morning to ensure that everyone running the race can be accounted for during the event. If a runner drops out, he or she must report to the finish line or to a safety official on the course so the course sweep doesn't have to search for a presumed-lost runner; unfortunately it is not uncommon for runners to check in at the start but never check back in at the finish line or elsewhere on the course. Safety personnel are then dispatched only to find the unaccounted-for runner back in the hotel, lounging by the pool.

Many of the entry-limit races such as the Mount Baldy Run Up in California (limit 600), the Tecumseh Trail Marathon (limit 700), and the Crazy Bob Bair Gutsman in Utah (limit 300) use the first-come, first-serve approach. Others, like the Mount Washington 7.6-Mile Hill Climb in Gorham, New Hampshire, use a lottery system for race entry. The majority of the 1,100 race slots are determined by a random draw, with a few reserved for elite or invited runners, the past year's award winners, any former race winner, and those with unbroken attendance streaks since 1984.

Some races reach entry limits by allowing only qualified participants an entry slot. This is most typical for 100-mile trail races and the most grueling of the shorter distance mountain races like the Escarpment 30K in New York's Catskill Mountains. The primary reason—safety. The U.S. Fila SkyMarathon in Aspen required participants to have finished a marathon or another high-altitude endurance event within 20 percent of the course record for entry consideration. Cutoff times are often instituted at various points along a course to further ensure safety for competitors and volunteers.

Some events reserve spots for top athletes, prior year volunteers, or very special cases. An alternative is to use a waiting list. Since 2000, organizers of the Pikes Peak Ascent and Marathon have placed athletes on a waiting list. Those athletes would have a shot at an entry slot only if cancellations occurred. The Leatherman's Loop Trail Race celebrated its 23rd running in 2009 and closed out at 1,200 entries in sixteen hours, and at least that many more put their names on a waiting list hoping to get in.

A creative approach for late entrants was started in the mid-1990s by the July Fourth Mount Marathon Race in Seward, Alaska. The night before the race during the bib number pickup, ten slots each in the men's and women's division of the race are auctioned. According to event organizers, "Competition is fierce, yet fun, with auction bids beginning at $75 and going as high as $1,175 for a single race slot."

Keep in mind that race directors often pad their limits, knowing that a percentage of runners won't show up on race day, typically 10 percent. Most races with entry limits accept no late entries period! If you plan to enter a trail or mountain race that has a published entry limit, it is best to contact race officials to make sure a space still exists. If the race director says the race is full, refrain from begging to be let in. Your case may be a special one; but be assured, many special cases arise, and race directors must draw the line somewhere. If the entry deadline was missed, request to be put on the mailing list for next year's event and make sure to get your entry in on time.

With the advent of online registration and sophisticated and interactive Web sites, event directors have been able to more closely monitor the influx of entries, and are better able to disseminate information on approaching entry limits with confirmed and potential entrants.

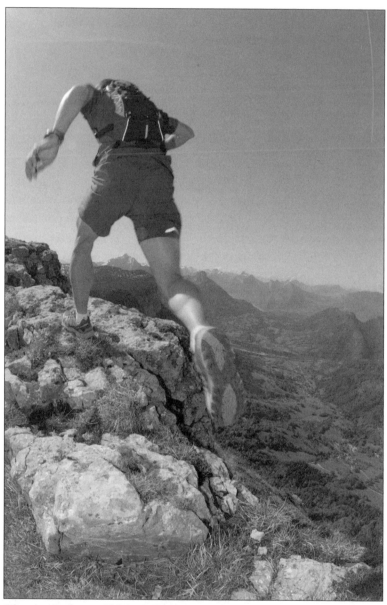

Often the view from up high is a trail runner's best prize. Stephan/Gripmaster

PERMITS AND RELATED ISSUES

As previously addressed, it is very likely that any course held on trails will require permits from the USDA Forest Service, parks department, governmental agency, or private land owner. Permits often require a detailed safety and communications plan, a course map, an entry form, a preliminary race budget, and an additional insured certificate. Some permitting agencies require that the event can only be put on by a 501(c)(3) (i.e., nonprofit) organization. If the event is being organized by a for-profit entity, race plans may be curtailed before the permit process begins. Be sure to secure all necessary permits (including insurance) for the race well in advance of the event, including both public and private land permits and/or written authorization. Part of the permit process may require posting signs at trailheads prior to and during the event, plus notifying via letters those residents living on or near land used or affected by the race. Following up with relevant agencies and individuals is imperative to ensure that all necessary requirements are fulfilled.

It is also a good idea to make friends with the permitting agencies or, better still, invite representatives from relevant agencies to sit on the organization committee and become involved with the event. Dale Garland directs the Hardrock 100 and maintains an open line of communication with the Bureau of Land Management and the USDA Forest Service. Garland involves the permit administrator in as much of the run as possible, from welcoming runners to working an aid station.

Making donations to the park (whether it is city, county, state, or federally owned and operated) or agency, or using your event as a fundraiser for a nonprofit group may also work in your favor. Brian Wieck directs the Pemberton Trail 50K in Fountain Hills, Arizona, where all park and permit fees are waived because proceeds from the race are donated back to the park. In order to stage the Mount Mitchell Challenge, Jim Curwen needed permission from nine different entities including the North Carolina State Parks, USDA Forest Service, National Park Service, two municipalities, a college, and three private landholder groups—one being a bear hunter's club. According to Curwen: "We not only received permission from those entities but have enjoyed their active support.

Why? We don't lie to them, we respect their rights, and we ask—not tell—them what we need. Most importantly, we say please and thank you."

Even if a permit is secured for an event, the issue of sharing the route with other multiuser groups may still arise. Most events do not close their courses to outside users. It is a good idea to befriend multiuser groups and perhaps ask them to volunteer or be supportive spectators on race day. Further, if the group's members provide volunteer support, offering the group a donation or getting trail runners to volunteer for their events will build goodwill.

COURSE LOGISTICS AND SUPPORT

Part of the safety plan should include aid or support stations on the course. Shorter duration events (those lasting under thirty minutes) require few or no aid stations, but they may require some support in terms of volunteers or medical assistance, depending on the terrain and potential for injuries. At minimum, water at the start/finish line and a first-aid kit should be available to competitors. Longer events require more and often different levels of aid, and USATF has come up with guidelines on what should be provided at aid stations. Remember that every course is different; some have more remote areas that make recruiting volunteer or even paid support difficult.

For some events supplies must be hauled to aid stations in unusual ways. The Kilauea Volcano Wilderness Marathon, last held in 2008, used horses and mules to haul supplies to three of their aid stations, and in the early years of the Pikes Peak Marathon a pack of llamas was enlisted for the same task. It is, however, recommended that trail runners become somewhat self-sufficient—even in the best-managed races—by carrying their own water and supplies to supplement what is provided on the course. Most important, whatever is promised to runners, make sure that it is delivered. If the entry form or course map states that six well-stocked aid stations are provided during the 25K, follow through by making sure aid is where it is supposed to be.

Aid that is part of the finish line setup should include some type of fluid replacement, be it water or an energy drink. Race timing should, of course, be located at the finish line, and if computerized scoring is selected, ensure access to power is readily available, which may require a generator if utilities are not within reach of an extension cord. Power will not be a concern if stopwatches or a Chronomix (a handheld battery-operated device) is used for timing. Chip timing has evolved over the past decade and can be most helpful in tracking runners at various points along a course, offering some great statistical data for race directors and runners who enjoy facts and figures. Chip timing is typically more expensive than standard clock timing, but not always. The recycling benefits of chip timing may outweigh the trash created from runner numbers and safety pins.

NAMING THE RACE

Event organization doesn't end with the course layout. The race director must also attend to promotions, marketing, typesetting, and printing. Promotion and marketing starts with the race name. The name may have been decided during the commitment phase of planning, or it may have evolved through the site selection phase, or during the choice of a race date. Many races include a cutoff time or the actual distance in the name, like the Anvil 59 Minute 39 Second Challenge in Nome, Alaska, 24 Hours of Frisco in Frisco, Colorado, or the Laurel Valley 34.7 Mile in Pickens, South Carolina. Seasons or temperatures are also common in race titles. November is the appropriate time for the After the Leaves Have Fallen Trail Run in New Paltz, New York, and August works for the Dog Days of Summer 8K in Arnold, Maryland.

It is also common to include the location of the race in the name, like the Bandera Trail Races, a 25K, 50K, and 100K in Bandera, Texas, or the Merrimack River Trail Run, a 10-miler held on the Merrimack River Trail in Andover, Massachusetts. The Dam Good Trail Run, a 20K in Mount Morris, New York, the Difficult Run Cross Country, an 8K in Great Falls, Virginia, the 7 Mile Ugly Mudder in Reading, Pennsylvania, and the Hernia Hill Half Marathon in Arnold, California, are names that are indicative of what might be encountered during the run. Sponsors of the race will benefit from increased publicity if their name is included in the event's title. Animals work in advertising spots on television and are often included in race titles to promote an event. There's the U Otter Run in Hudson,

Illinois, the Rattlesnake Ramble in Eldorado Canyon, Colorado, and the Muddy Moose Trail Race in Wolfeboro, New Hampshire.

After researching more than 800 trail race names, the most common words used in titles are *wild, mountain, classic, challenge,* and *adventure* with *trail* being the clear favorite, with more than 300 using it. However, trail racers should be forewarned that not all races with the term trail in the title are off-road events. If unfamiliar with a particular event, the best way to ensure that the event is indeed an off-road trail race is to contact the race director to get a full course description before registering.

ENTRY FORMS AND ENTRY FEES

The entry form is one of the most important documents for the event, and it should be used as an educational tool for prospective runners as well as a marketing and promotional avenue for the media and sponsors. Whether the entry form is hard copy or posted online, information should be readable and complete, with the following information bold-faced or highlighted: name of the race, date, start time and location, course description, and contact information for further details. A liability waiver should be included on the entry form and/or be made available for signature at packet pickup. Keep on file all completed liability waivers for reference should a claim be filed by a participant. Laws vary from state to state as to the length of time waivers need to be kept on file. Legal assistance can be sought to draft an appropriate waiver, or an insurance company can be contacted to supply a sample waiver. Be sure that the insurance company providing insurance coverage for the race reviews the waiver to ensure that it complies with the terms of the insurance package. If liability waivers are not collected from participants until race day, long lines may ensue. On the other hand, collection on race day ensures that everyone checked in and an accurate count of all runners competing will be forthcoming. Although computer chip timing is an alternative for quick check-in, it is usually too costly for small events.

As mentioned previously, a detailed course description is a must in the entry materials. Not only will this minimize calls or e-mails to the race director, but it also enables runners to find the route and train in advance of the event. Be specific about the terrain and potential hazards that may exist on the route. Include a map of the course. The map should be hand drawn or be represented on a topographic map. It is very helpful to create a course profile including overall ascent and descent as well as average grade. Indicate where the aid/support stations are and what facilities runners will find at the various aid stations. Offer clothing suggestions for expected as well as unexpected weather conditions; advise runners as to potential weather extremes and include the average temperatures for the time period.

The entry form should solicit basic runner participant information: name, address, age and birthdate, gender, e-mail address, and an emergency contact. If space allows, gather biographical information on the entrant's trail running experience, and provide this to the race announcer and for media releases. If the race requires specific qualifications, like completing a marathon or racing at high altitude, the registration form should request such information.

Many items already discussed require a fee and should be itemized in the race budget. A race budget is key to successful financial planning. The established entry fee determines a lot of race amenities. Conversely, total projected expenses may dictate the entry fee. The race director or race committee can base the entry fee on comparable events, or include expenses in a preliminary budget and calculate the necessary entry fee to defray those costs. Don't be surprised to learn that more money may be required than is reasonable to charge in an entry fee to break even. On the other hand, some costs normally associated with road races (like police and expensive computerized timing) may not apply to trail races. Be sure the entry fee fairly reflects what the event promises to deliver—the view alone may be priceless, but the event still needs to provide amenities that correspond with the dollar amount charged to each participant.

AWARDS

Choosing awards can be a challenge for even the most creative race director. Although most runners have lots of T-shirts, this is still the most common item runners receive for their race entry fee. A one-size-fits-all item such as a hat, cowbell, or a bag makes good sense and certainly streamlines ordering as it eliminates the need for small-medium-large-extra large size estimates. Remember that you can use items year after year as long as the date isn't screened or embroidered on the item.

For race prizes, consider first the awards structure. Some event directors give an award or memento to each finisher. This might be a T-shirt that is embossed with "finisher" above or below a race logo, or perhaps a medal inscribed with the word "finisher." The Laurel Highlands Ultra finisher award is a miniature version of the little concrete pillar mileage marker.

Finisher awards may indicate a competitor's time, like those of the Leadville Trail 100 where finishers under twenty-five hours receive a large, handcrafted gold and silver trophy belt buckle and finishers under thirty hours receive a handcrafted silver belt buckle. All women finishers under thirty hours at Leadville also receive a gold and silver pendant.

Some events award prizes to just the top finisher overall in the male and female divisions, while others choose to award the top three, the top five, or in some cases, the top ten. Age group division prizes typically range from five- to ten-year increments and may be presented to the top finisher in each category, or perhaps the top five per category depending on the number of finishers expected in each category.

Some awards earn a special place on the mantle, while others may sit in a box. Favorite prizes are often those that elicit a favorite memory from a race.

Englishman Paul Bateson, who now conducts events in his adopted home of Spain, recalls his most memorable prize, a bronze model of the race route. Jonathan Beverly got a slice of a tree trunk with a plaque affixed to it for winning the 1991 York Gulch Trail Race in St. Mary's Glacier in Idaho Springs, Colorado. Andrew Fairhurst recalls a gold coin he won for the Canadian Death Race in 2005. Fellow Canadian Pam Pedlow, who has been running trails since 1975, recalls her best prize in a trail race: "It has to be my Indian carving I received for placing first in my age group in the Knee Knackering North Shore 50K Trail Run in 2003. Another good one was a mounted rock from the inaugural Dirty Duo 25K."

One of Annette Bednosky's most coveted awards is the bronze-casted cougar trophy she received for her win at the 2005 Western States

100. "I put it in my carry-on luggage and it became a novelty in airport security. From behind me a pilot—an ultrarunner—recognized the cougar as the prize for winning WS 100. His surprise and congratulations were hearty and extensive, drawing attention from other passengers as he explained the significance. It was the best time I ever had going through airport security. The cougar now lives on the floor of our living room."

A prize may not always be a favorite, but rather enjoyed for its uniqueness, like the rubber chicken Scott Dunlap won at the Golden Gate Headlands Marathon.

Prizes may be functional like clothing or decorative like ceramic pottery, or even flowers for a garden. David Wise from Hyde Park, New York, once received a flat of petunias for finishing second in his age group in a race in Poughkeepsie, New York.

Still other prizes may be in the form of food or drink. The most memorable prize Rickey Gates says he won was a 6-liter bottle of champagne from a race in Slovenia. "It seemed preposterous to carry it around with me on my touring bicycle from race to race so I asked my friend Anna Pichrtova to take it for me. She traveled with it through four countries where it ended up in Switzerland for post-race festivities (at the 2008 World Mountain Running Championships)."

Paul Horstmann of Pleasant Valley, New York, recalls winning a box of dessert confections including éclairs and Napoleons. New Zealander Paul Charteris won 50 kilograms of maize at Mexico's Copper Canyon Ultramarathon, which he donated to the Raramuri people of Batopilas.

Whatever the awards, be sure to advertise what runners can expect and also whether they must be in attendance at the awards ceremony to receive their prizes, or whether they will be mailed or available for pickup after the event. If an event director plans an enjoyable post-race celebration or random prize giveaways, runners may be more inclined to stick around for the awards. Perhaps Americans can learn something from the Europeans, whose post-event celebrations are renowned for often lasting well into the evening. Rickey Gates, mentioned above, often spends summers racing in Europe and enjoys the pre- and post-race atmosphere as well as the good competition. In fact Gates says it was summed up for him by an Austrian race director, who "late in the evening wrapped his massive trunk of an arm around me sloshing wine all about and said, 'You know what I love about you guys? Before the race you are friends, after the race you are drinking friends, but during the race, *how you fight!!*'"

CANCELLATION DUE TO WEATHER

Trail races, like road races, are typically held regardless of rain, shine, sleet, or snow. However, the chance always exists that some unexpected natural hazard such as an earthquake, tornado, forest fire, extreme temperature change, mudslide, substantial accumulation of snow, lightning, or avalanche may force cancellation, delay, or postponement of the event. Of primary concern is the safety of race participants and volunteers on the course. The race director should evaluate every hazard, real and potential, on a case-by-case basis because no clear rules exist regarding cancellation or postponement of events. Ultimately, the race director (with input from the race committee) will make the final determination whether to stage the event. Have an alternate plan that addresses the potential postponement, delay, shortening the race distance, or cancellation of the event, and if you adopt such a plan, be sure the new information can be relayed to runners in a timely fashion.

BANDITS

The biggest nemesis for race directors is the bandit. Although participation by non-entrants may seem innocent enough to other runners, they are the bane of race directors, especially when bandits use amenities at aid stations and post-race refreshment tables. Characterizing these runners as bandits is appropriate because they are robbing the race, taking something that they didn't pay for by enjoying refreshments, getting a finish time, cruising along on a well-marked course, and availing themselves of the potential assistance of medical staff.

In backcountry trail events, particularly those held on extreme courses, bandits are a threat to their own safety and that of registered entrants. Trail, mountain, and adventure races occur in remote areas and require dedicated volunteers and mountain rescue workers to assist in the case of injuries, lost racers, or extreme weather. Because bandits are not registered, they do not check into or out of aid stations. They do, unfortunately, take supplies from such stations, and it is not unheard of for a back-of-the-pack ultrarunner to arrive at a remote aid station that has been left dry because unofficial runners have depleted it of liquids or energy bars.

Concerted efforts on the part of paying registered participants to discourage and report bandits will have a positive impact. Race directors can notify potential bandits with warning statements in race information: "Warning—those found on the course without proof of official entry will be tarred, feathered, and immediately expunged from further participation!" Pre-race announcements can also strongly urge bandits to go for a training run on another route.

DIRECTING A TRAIL/MOUNTAIN RACE—TIMELINE

The following suggestions should be modified to suit a particular event.

At Least Twelve Months before Race

- Recruit race committee and/or key officers and stage an initial organizational meeting.

- Make a mental commitment to do the event after thoughtful consideration and goal setting, often an offshoot of the initial organizational meeting.

- Select site/venue.

- Select distance(s).

- Select race name.

- Select date and time, checking calendar (other running event calendars in your region) to avoid conflicts.

- Obtain written permissions to use land and facilities; apply and pay for all necessary permits.

- Prepare preliminary budget for the event.

- Prepare preliminary duty roster for key positions within the race organization.

- Measure course(s) and create a course profile map.

- Secure Web site—either existing or create one, and consider social networking through Facebook, Twitter, etc.

- Open checking account for all transactions related to the event (incoming registrations, sponsor donations, outgoing bills).

- Develop operations manual or notebook to keep paperwork in order.

Six to Twelve Months before Race

- Obtain insurance and additional insured certificate for any agencies that require one.

- Draft a race logo with the aid of a graphic designer or a creative volunteer.

- Begin mailings for inclusion in annual calendars (magazines, chambers of commerce/visitor bureaus, local newspapers) and prepare advance press release for publicity.

- Secure, if possible, a list of potential runners to contact via e-mail with details on the event. Lists may be available for purchase or rental from other events or clubs for a one-time use. A running store may be willing to provide an e-mail list in exchange for a sponsor mention.

- Prepare the race entry form and make a list of distribution centers that includes health clubs, specialty running stores, sporting good retailers, colleges, and large corporations.

- Contact a registration service to make the entry form available online.

- Set up a schedule for race committee meetings—monthly to begin with and more frequently as the event nears. Prepare a meeting agenda, stick to it, and try to finish your meetings within one hour.

- Identify potential sponsors (in-kind and cash), then approach and secure sponsors.

- Obtain commitment for help for key positions (timing, results, aid, etc.) and assign tasks.

- Start processing entries received.

At Least Six Months before Race

- Order or obtain source for supplies (runner race numbers, pins, cups, additional merchandise for sale, etc.). Seek competitive bids—up to three is standard. Some supplies may be in-kind product donations that will help to offset budgeted expense items. Where possible use recycled items and prepare for and provide recycling options on race day.

- Confirm sources for and order special equipment:
  - Safety—walkie-talkies, cell phones, ambulance, search and rescue teams
  - Comfort—portable toilets (rule of thumb is 1:100 runners for large events; 1:50 for smaller events)
  - Course—flagging/flour, snow groomer, tape, cones, banners; again consider recyclable/green materials for all course markings
  - Awards—bibs, race T-shirts, prizes, random prizes

- Hold an organizational meeting with key players, and produce a list of all contacts with phone, fax, and e-mail. Prepare an agenda and keep both agenda and meeting notes on file for future reference and planning.

One to Four Months before Race

- Finalize key volunteer positions.

- Set event specifics (exact route, power needs at start/finish, fee, etc.).

- Continue entry form distribution. Exposure on social networking sites is also suggested.

- Circulate press releases announcing the event and look for and share special interest stories with the media—think both news and feature.

- Conduct organizational meetings as necessary.

Two to Four Weeks before Race

- Make follow-up phone calls to media (those to whom press materials were sent).

- Have equipment, prizes, supplies on hand—be sure to inventory the items and test all equipment for working order.

- Remind key volunteers of their duties (provide them with a checklist), and give them additional written instructions and/or meet with people to go over the plan.

- Notify local emergency agencies and medical volunteers (fire, ambulance, etc.) of the event and route.

One Week before Race

- Inspect route and modify as required (weather, terrain/erosion).

- Process pre-registrations and assign bib numbers.

- Post any signage about the event to alert other trail users in advance.

- Assemble event packets.

Final Week

- Continue entry processing.

- Assemble all supplies.

- Firmly tie up loose ends.

Day before Race

- Mark route, inspect area.

- Hold pre-race meeting, if one has been scheduled for competitors (make this decision early on).

Day of Race

- Make sure all volunteers are in place.

- Put up banners and start/finish line.

- Inspect *all* course markings prior to the competitors starting out on the course. Have a broom, rake, and/or shovel at the start if necessary to clean away debris.

- Make preliminary race announcements.

- Make sure timing devices are working.

- Start the race *on time*.

- Clean and sweep route after the last competitor finishes.

- Remove and dispose of all trash.

- Stage the awards ceremony.

- Furnish press release with results and photos to media ASAP by e-mail.

- Send results to participants via Internet or e-mail, and post in local running stores (either race day or within one week following the event).

- Incorporate digital photos to accompany press releases. Share all the news with your sponsors.

Day After

- Remove remaining course markings, clean and clear any traces of event.

- Follow up with media.

- Tie up any loose ends.

Two Days After

- *Rest,* but start thinking about next year's event!

Week After

- Hold wrap-up meeting with volunteers and officials—encourage feedback and criticism and how event can be improved next year. Mail thank-you letters to sponsors, permitees, helpers, others.

- Store and return necessary equipment.

- Write down ideas for next year and start working on them!

CHECKLIST

Committee Assignments

These are some key areas of responsibility—depending on the size of the race, one individual may take on more than one area of responsibility.

- race director

- course director

- equipment director

- medical and emergency facilities director

- sponsor liaison

- press director

- communications director

- awards/prizes

- registrar

- treasurer

- merchandise sales

- finish line

- timing/scoring

- webmaster

Supplies

- Aid station—First-aid kit, water, cups, energy drinks, bars, gels (dictated by time/distance of event), runner registration list (both alpha and numeric), communication equipment (radio, CB, cell phone—check range of cell phone prior to race day)

- Course—markings to include flour or flagging, duct tape, clipboards, banners, rope, and twisty ties (for banners)

- Registration—credit card machine, change (one- or five-dollar bills), pens, pencils, markers, safety pins, runner numbers, entry forms including liability waivers

- Finish line—banners, chutes, flour line across the trail, copy of all permits required to stage the race

- Timing equipment—clipboards, stopwatch, Chronomix, race clock

Race Packets

- Course map

- Sponsor materials—product or printed materials

- Coupons

- Race rules

- Runner survey to get feedback from the participants. You can also put the survey online.

SAMPLE PRESS RELEASE

July 20, 2009

For Immediate Release

Contact: Nancy Hobbs (719) 573-4133 or trlrunner@aol.com

Colorado Springs, Colorado—On Sunday, July 26, trail and mountain running enthusiasts will gather at the start line in North Cheyenne Cañon to enjoy the trails and open spaces afforded by the area, including ascents, rolling hills, and a variety of terrain underfoot.

The Cheyenne Cañon Mountain Race, presented by Walmart, is a first-year event and will offer an 8K course for open women, junior women, and junior men and a 12K course for open men.

The competitors will include the nation's best mountain runners who will vie for spots on the 2009 Teva U.S. Mountain Running Team, which will compete in Campodolcino, Italy, this September. "This event is the second and final selection race for the team, and the course mirrors the World Championships course in Italy," said race director Nancy Hobbs.

The event will start with the women running at 7:00 a.m. and the men following at 8:30 a.m. There is a limited race field with 100 entries per gender.

Proceeds from the event will be distributed between the following 501(c)(3) nonprofits: the American Trail Running Association, Friends of North Cheyenne Cañon, and Stratton Commons.

Additional race sponsors include Marzolf-Blessing/ERA Shields, Dr. Matthews with Champion Health, Teva, SportHill, Colorado Running Company, and Criterium Bike Shops.

For more information visit www.trailrunner.com.

SAMPLE RACE BUDGET

Expense Category

- advertising
- aid station supplies
- awards
- awards—prize money
- communications
- copies
- donation/charitable giving
- first-aid kits
- insurance
- medical/ambulance
- office supplies
- permits
- portable toilets
- postage
- printing brochures
- results
- runner numbers
- sanction fees
- scoring/timing
- T-shirts
- Web site

Total Expenses:

Income Category

- donations

- entry fees—mail-in/online

- sponsorships

- merchandise sales

Total Income:

Net Income:

APPENDIX:
COMPETING AT THE INTERNATIONAL LEVEL

Since 1985, the WMRA, formerly the International Committee on Mountain Running (ICMR), has hosted the annual World Mountain Trophy Race—name changed to World Mountain Running Championships starting in 2009—which is usually held during the first or second week of September. The events are administered under patronage of the IAAF and include senior men, senior women, junior men, and junior women competitions and usually an open race for citizen runners. For junior competition an athlete must be at least sixteen but not yet twenty in the year of competition. All those twenty and above on December 31 in the year of competition are eligible for the senior competition. There is no maximum age limit for seniors.

In order to accommodate two forms of mountain running, the World Mountain Running Championships is held on European-style uphill courses in even-numbered years and up/down courses in odd-numbered years to mirror the British version. Distances vary, but typically senior men run a 12K course, senior women and junior men run an 8K route, while junior women run approximately 4.5K. Awards are presented to the top three individuals as well as the top three teams in each category. A separate masters (age forty and above) competition is not associated with the championship race, but an open race that includes age-group divisions is typically scheduled during the weekend activities. No prize money is awarded to top finishers, and each country or, in some cases, the athletes themselves must pay travel expenses to the host venue. However, the host country supplies meals and lodging for participants during the three- to four-day stay during the events.

In order for a country's athletes to compete on the international level in IAAF-recognized events, including the IAAF World Cross Country Championships, World Mountain Running Championships events, and the 100K World Challenge (a road event), a nation's governing body must be a member association of the international body. For the United States that organization is USATF.

The United States has competed in the mountain championships since 1989, fielding a full senior men's team starting in 1992 and a full senior women's team since 1995. The United States added juniors to their squad in 2003. Up to thirty-six countries participate in the championships each year. U.S. athletes can earn a berth on the national team by posting a top finish in one of the selection races usually held in June or July. The Mountain Ultra Trail (MUT) Council awards the selection races at the annual USATF convention through a bid process. Additional team members are selected based on their race results from mountain, trail, and road races as well as past performances in international competitions including the World Championships. Athletes representing the United States must be current members of USATF.

The WMRA developed a grand prix mountain running series that includes annually between five and seven events, most often with venues in Europe and the United Kingdom, held during the spring and summer. Interested nations must present a bid for series designation and pay a fee to the WMRA. Each event is held independently, with points as well as prize money being awarded to the top finishers. Series champions that are determined at the end of the season receive additional awards and prize money. The WMRA also oversees the World Youth Championship and the World Mountain Running Masters Championships annually, and the WMRA World Long Distance Mountain Running Challenge, which is an event staged as part of an existing event (for instance, the Jungfrau Marathon and Pikes Peak Marathon have both hosted the event), providing WMRA medals to the top finishers.

There were seven events in the 2009 Skyrunner World Series and nine events in the Skyrunner World Series Trials from which athletes could garner points. Skyrunner World Series races are open to individual Skyrunners and sponsored teams based on the sum of the best three World Series results and one World Series Trial. (Double points are awarded at the final to the top fifteen ranked men and top eight ranked women). Team points are not awarded in the World Series Trials. The final prize purse in 2009 was €10,000. The United States presently offers one event on the Skyrunning calendar, but in the future may include more events. Contact www.skyrunning.com for more information.

BIBLIOGRAPHY

Anderson, Bob. *Stretching,* rev. ed. Bolinas, CA: Shelter Publications, 2000.

Armstrong, Lawrence E., PhD. *Performing in Extreme Environments.* Champaign, IL: Human Kinetics Publishers, 2000.

Bernardot, Dan, PhD, RD. *Nutrition for Serious Athletes.* Champaign, IL: Human Kinetics Publishers, 2000.

Benyo, Richard, ed. *Marathon & Beyond,* Champaign, IL: 42K(+) Press.

Burke, Ed R., PhD. *Cycling Health and Physiology: Using Sports Science to Improve Your Riding and Racing.* College Park, MD: Vitesse Press, 1998.

Burke, Ed R., PhD. *Optimal Muscle Recovery.* Wayne, NJ: Avery Publishing Group, Inc., 1999.

Clark, Nancy, MS, RD. *Nancy Clark's Sports Nutrition Guidebook.* Champaign, IL: Human Kinetics Publishers, 1997.

Craythorn, Dennis, and Rich Hanna. *The Ultimate Runner's Journal: Your Daily Training Partner and Log.* Marathon Publishers, Inc., 1998.

Daniels, Jack, PhD. *Daniels' Formula.* Champaign, IL: Human Kinetics Publishers, 1998.

Dorfman, Lisa, MS, RD, LHMC. *The Vegetarian Sports Nutrition Guide: Peak Performance for Everyone from Beginners to Gold Medalists.* New York: Wiley, 2000.

Forgey, William, MD. *Wilderness Medicine,* 4th ed. Oakland, CA: ICS Books, 1994.

Gastelu, Daniel, and Dr. Fred Hatfield. *Dynamic Nutrition for Maximum Performance.* Wayne, NJ: Avery Publishing Group, 1997.

Girard-Eberle, Suzanne. *Endurance Sports Nutrition.* Champaign, IL: Human Kinetics Publishers, 2000.

Haas, Dr. Robert. *Eat to Win: The Sports Nutrition Bible.* New York: Rawson Associates, 1983.

Hanc, John. *The Essential Runner.* New York: The Lyons Press, 1994.

Johnson, Joan M. *The Healing Art of Sports Massage.* Emmaus, PA: Rodale Press, 1995.

McAtee, Robert E., and Jeff Charland. *Facilitated Stretching.* Champaign, IL: Human Kinetics Publishers, 2007.

McQuaide, Mike. *Trail Running Guide to Western Washington.* Seattle, WA: Sasquatch Books, 2001.

Mislinski, Phil, Monique Cole, and Scott Boulbol. *Trail Runner's Guide to Colorado: 50 Great Trail Runs.* Golden, CO: Fulcrum Publishing, 1999.

Murray, Frank. *Happy Feet.* New Canaan, CT: Keats Publishing, Inc., 1993.

Null, Gary, and Dr. Howard Robins. *Ultimate Training: Gary Null's Complete Guide to Eating Right, Exercise, and Living Longer.* New York: St. Martin's Press, 1993.

Peterson, Marilyn S. *A Guide to Sports Nutrition: Eat to Compete.* Saint Louis, MO: Mosby, 1996.

Runner's World magazine, Emmaus, PA: Rodale, www.runnersworld.com

Running Times magazine, Wilton, CT: www.runningtimes.com

Sandrock, Michael. *Running Tough: 75 Challenging Training Runs.* Champaign, IL: Human Kinetics Publishers, 2001.

Spitz, Barry. *Dipsea: The Greatest Race.* San Anselmo, CA: Potrero Meadow Publishing Co., 1993.

Swartz, Stan, James W. Wolff, and Samir Shahin. *50 Trail Runs in Southern California.* Seattle: Mountaineers Books, 2000.

The Running Times Guide to Breakthrough Running, Champaign, IL: Human Kinetics Publishers, 2000.

Trail Runner Magazine, Boulder, CO: North South Publications. www.trailrunnermag.com

UltraRunning magazine, Healdsburg, CA. www.ultrarunning.com

INDEX

ABOUT THE AUTHORS

Adam W. Chase grew up running trails in Colorado and Vermont, and has since gone on to run hundreds of races throughout much of the world as a sponsored trail and ultrarunner, adventure racer, and snowshoe racer. He is also the Trail Editor of *Running Times* and has contributed to *Trail Runner, Ultrarunning, Outside, Marathon & Beyond, Competitor,* and *Runner's World,* among others. Chase is a proud father of two sons and lives in Boulder, Colorado.

Nancy Hobbs has been running trails and directing running events since the mid-80s, and her articles and photographs have been published in magazines including *Trail Runner, Ultrarunning, Running Times,* and *Runner's World.* She is the founder and executive director of the American Trail Running Association, a council member of the World Mountain Running Association, manager of the Teva U.S. Mountain Running Team, and chairperson of the USATF Mountain Ultra Trail Council. She lives in Colorado Springs.